THEN AGAIN

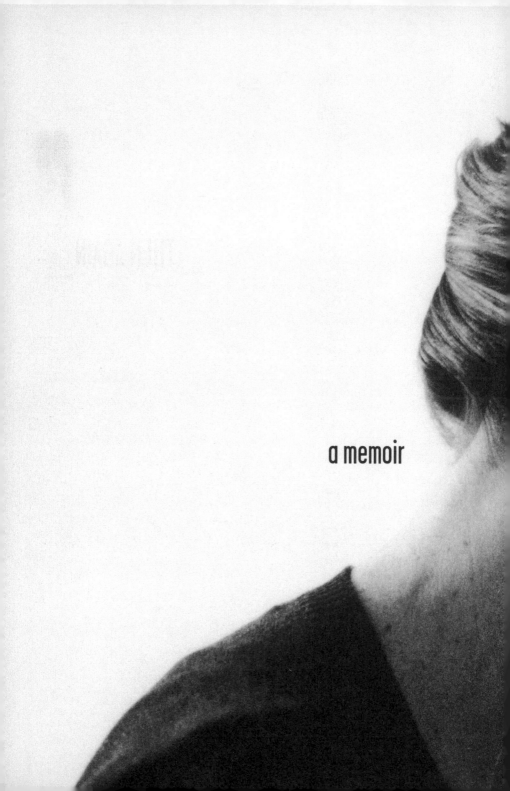

a memoir

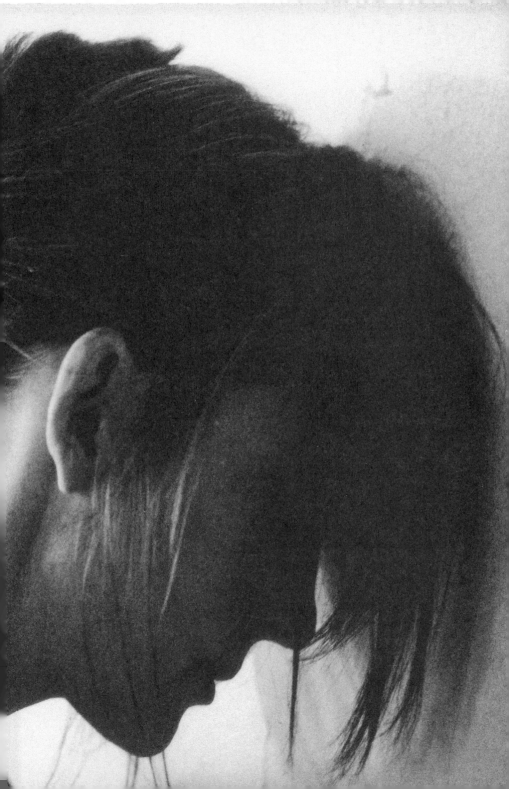

THEN AGAIN

DIANE KEATON

RANDOM HOUSE
NEW YORK

Then Again is a work of nonfiction. Some names and
identifying details have been changed.

Copyright © 2011 by Diane Keaton

All rights reserved.

Published in the United States by Random House, an imprint of
The Random House Publishing Group, a division of
Random House, Inc., New York.

RANDOM HOUSE and colophon are registered trademarks
of Random House, Inc.

Quote from *Annie Hall* copyright © 1977 by Metro Goldwyn Mayer.
All rights reserved. Used by permission.

Quotes from the Lincoln Center Tribute for Diane Keaton speech
by Woody Allen copyright © 2007 by Woody Allen.
All other text by Woody Allen copyright © 2011 by Woody Allen.
Used by permission.

Credits for photographs and artwork
appear on pages 263–65.

LIBRARY OF CONGRESS CATALOGING-IN-PUBLICATION DATA
Keaton, Diane.
Then again / by Diane Keaton.
p.   cm.
ISBN 978-1-4000-6878-4
eBook ISBN 978-1-58836-942-0
1. Keaton, Diane. 2. Keaton, Diane—Family. 3. Motion picture actors and
actresses—United States—Biography. I. Title.
PN2287.K44A3 2011
791.43'028092—dc23   2011023752
[B]

Printed in the United States of America on acid-free paper

www.atrandom.com

2 4 6 8 9 7 5 3 1

First Edition

Book design by Emily Harwood Blass

To my City of Women:

Stephanie Heaton, Sandra Shadic, Lindsay Dwelley.
Plus two men: David Ebershoff and Bill Clegg.
They know why.

I always say my life is this family, and that's the truth.
Dorothy Deanne Keaton Hall

THINK

Mom loved adages, quotes, slogans. There were always little reminders pasted on the kitchen wall. For example, the word THINK. I found THINK thumbtacked on a bulletin board in her darkroom. I saw it Scotch-taped on a pencil box she'd collaged. I even found a pamphlet titled THINK on her bedside table. Mom liked to THINK. In a notebook she wrote, *I'm reading Tom Robbins's book* Even Cowgirls Get the Blues. *The passage about marriage ties in with women's struggle for accomplishment. I'm writing this down for future THINKING . . .* She followed with a Robbins quote: *"For most poor dumb brainwashed women marriage is the climactic experience. For men, marriage is a matter of efficient logistics: the male gets his food, bed, laundry, TV . . . offspring and creature comforts all under one roof. . . . But for a woman, marriage is surrender. Marriage is when a girl gives up the fight . . . and from then on leaves the truly inter-*

esting and significant action to her husband, who has bar-
gained to 'take care' of her. . . . Women live longer than men
because they really haven't been living." Mom liked to THINK
about life, especially the experience of being a woman. She
liked to write about it too.

In the mid-seventies on a visit home, I was printing some
photographs I'd taken of Atlantic City in Mother's darkroom when I found something I'd never seen. It was some
kind of, I don't know, sketchbook. On the cover was a collage she'd made out of family photographs with the words
It's the Journey That Counts, Not the Arrival. I picked it up
and flipped through the pages. Although it included several
collages made from snapshots and magazine cutouts, it was
filled with page after page of writing.

Had a productive day at Hunter's Bookstore. We re-
arranged the art section and discovered many interesting
books hidden away. It's been two weeks since I was hired.
I make 3 dollars and thirty-five cents an hour. Today I got
paid 89 dollars in total.

This wasn't one of Mom's typical scrapbooks, with the
usual napkins from Clifton's Cafeteria, old black-and-white
photographs, and my less-than-thrilling report cards. This
was a journal.

An entry dated August 2, 1976, read: WATCH OUT
ON THIS PAGE. *For you, the possible reader in the future,*
this takes courage. I'm speaking of what is on my mind. I
am angry. Target—Jack—bad names, those he has flung
at me—NOT forgotten and that is undoubtedly the
problem—"You frigin' bastard"—all said—all felt. God,
who the hell does he think he is?

That was it for me. This was raw, too raw. I didn't want to know about an aspect of Mother and Father's life that could shatter my perception of their love. I put it down, walked out of the darkroom, and did not open another one of her eighty-five journals until she died some thirty years later. But, of course, no matter how hard I tried to deny their presence, I couldn't help but see them resting on bookshelves, or placed underneath the telephone, or even staring up at me from inside a kitchen drawer. One time I began looking through Mom's new Georgia O'Keeffe *One Hundred Flowers* picture book on the coffee table, only to find a journal titled *Who Says You Haven't Got a Chance?* lying underneath. It was as if they were conspiring, "Pick us up, Diane. Pick us up." Forget it. There was no way I was going to go through that experience again. But I was impressed with Mom's tenacity. How could she keep writing without an audience, not even her own family? She just did.

She wrote about going back to school at age forty. She wrote about being a teacher. She wrote about every stray cat she rescued. When her sister Marti got skin cancer and lost most of her nose, she wrote about that too. She wrote about her frustrations with aging. When Dad got sick in 1990, her journal raged at the injustice of the cancer that attacked his brain. The documentation of his passing proved to be some of Mom's finest reporting. It was as if taking care of Jack made her love him in a way that helped her become the person she always wished she could have been.

I was trying to get Jack to eat today. But he couldn't. After a while, I took off my glasses. I put my head close to his, and I told him, I whispered to him, that I missed him. I started to cry. I didn't want him to see, so I turned my head away. And Jack, with what little strength remained in that damn body of his, took a napkin from my pocket and slowly, as with everything he did, slowly, so slowly, he looked at me with those piercing blue eyes and wiped the tears away from my face. "We'll make it through this, Dorothy."

He didn't. In the end, Mom took care of Dad, just as she had taken care of Randy, Robin, Dorrie, and me—all our lives. But who was there for her when she wrote in a shaky hand: *June 1993. This is the day I heard I have the beginning of Alzheimer's disease. Scary.* Thus began a fifteen-year battle against the loss of memory.

She kept writing. When she could no longer write paragraphs, she wrote sentences like *Would we hurt each other less if we touched each other more?* and *Honor thyself.* And short questions and statements like *Quick. What's today's date?* Or odd things like *My head is taking a turn.* When she couldn't write sentences, she wrote words: *RENT. CALL. FLOWERS. CAR.* And even her favorite word, *THINK.* When she ran out of words, she wrote numbers, until she couldn't write anymore.

Dorothy Deanne Keaton was born in Winfield, Kansas, in 1921. Her parents, Beulah and Roy, drifted into California before she was three. They were heartlanders in search of the big dream. It dumped them into the hills of Pasadena. Mom played the piano and sang in a trio called Two Dots and a Dash at her high school. She was sixteen when her father drove off, leaving Beulah and her three daughters to fend for themselves. It was hard times for the Keaton girls in the late thirties. Beulah, who'd never worked a day in her life, had to find a job. Dorothy gave up her college dreams in order to help around the house until Beulah finally found work as a janitor.

I have a photograph of sixteen-year-old Dorothy standing next to her father, Roy Keaton. Why did he leave his favorite daughter, his look-alike; why? How could he have driven away knowing he would forever break some part of her heart?

Everything changed when Dorothy met Jack Hall on a basketball court at Los Angeles Pacific College in Highland Park. Mom loved to recall how this handsome black-haired, blue-eyed young man had come to meet her sister Martha but only had eyes for her. She would laugh and say, "It was love at first sight." And it must have been, because not long after that, they eloped in Las Vegas at the Stardust Hotel.

Mother never told me of her dreams for herself. There were hints though. She was president of the PTA as well as the Arroyo Vista Ladies Club. She was a Sunday-school teacher at our Free Methodist church. She entered every contest on the back of every cereal box. She loved game shows. Our favorite was *Queen for a Day,* emceed by Jack Bailey, who began each episode, five days a week, with "Would YOU like to be . . . QUEEN . . . FOR . . . A . . . DAY?" The game went like this: Bailey interviewed four women; whoever was in the worst shape—assessed by the audience applause meter—was crowned Queen for a Day. With "Pomp and Circumstance" playing, he would wrap the winner in a velvet cape with a white fur collar, place a sparkling tiara on her head, and give her four dozen red coronation roses from

Carl's of Hollywood. Mom and Auntie Martha wrote their sad stories on the application sheet more than once. She almost made the cut when she wrote, "My husband needs a lung." When pressed for details, Mom told the truth—well, sort of. Jack Hall, an ardent skin diver, needed to dive deeper in order to put more food on his family's plates. Mom was eliminated.

One morning I woke up to a group of strangers walking around our house examining every room. Mom hadn't bothered to tell us she had entered the Mrs. America contest at our local level. Mrs. America was a pageant devoted to finding the ideal homemaker. Later she informed us kids it was a competition of skills that included table-setting, floral-arranging, bed-making, and cooking, as well as managing the family budget and excelling in personal grooming. All we could think was WOW.

I was nine, so that made me old enough to sit in the audience of the movie theater on Figueroa Street when she was crowned Mrs. Highland Park. Suddenly my mother, the new greatest homemaker in Highland Park, stood high above me on a vast stage in front of a huge red velvet curtain. When the drapery opened to reveal an RCA Victor Shelby television, a Philco washer and dryer, a set of Samsonite luggage, a fashion wardrobe from Ivers Department Store, and six cobalt-blue flasks filled with Evening in Paris perfume, I wasn't sure what I was looking at. What was I seeing? Why was Mom standing in the spotlight like she was some sort of movie star? This was terribly exciting yet extremely unpleasant at the same time. Something had happened, a kind of betrayal. Mom had abandoned me, but, even worse, much worse, I secretly wished it would have been me on that stage, not her.

Six months later Dorothy Hall was crowned again, this time as Mrs. Los Angeles by Art Linkletter at the Ambassador Hotel. My brother, Randy, and I watched on the new RCA Victor Shelby television. Her duties as Mrs. Los Angeles included making local appearances at supermarkets, department stores, and ladies' clubs all over Los Angeles County. She wasn't home much, and when she was, she was busy baking the same German chocolate cake with walnuts over and over, in hopes she would be crowned Mrs. California. Dad got sick of the whole ordeal and made it known. When she lost the coveted title of Mrs. California, she appeared to accept her failure as easily as she resumed her normal household duties, but things were different, at least for me.

Sometimes I wonder how our lives might have changed if Mother had been chosen Mrs. America. Would she have become a TV personality like Bess Myerson, or a spokesperson for Philco appliances, or a columnist for *McCall's* magazine? What would have happened to my dreams of being in the spotlight if hers had been realized? Another mother took her opportunity away, but I didn't care; I was glad I didn't have to share her with a larger world.

Mom believed her kids would have brilliant futures. After all, I was funny. Randy wrote poems. Robin sang, and Dorrie was smart. By the time I was in junior high school, enough C-minuses had accumulated to prove I wasn't going to be a student with a brilliant future. Like the rest of the nation, I was tested for my intelligence in 1957. The results were not surprising. There was one exception, something called Abstract Reasoning. I couldn't wait to run home and tell Mom about this Abstract Reasoning thing. What was it? Excited by any accomplishment, she told me abstract reasoning was the ability to analyze information and solve problems on a complex, thought-based level. No matter how hard I've tried to figure out answers to problems by thinking them through, I still don't exactly understand what abstract reasoning means.

In 1959 our family's cultural outlook changed when the Bastendorfs moved next door. Bill was a psychologist, with a PhD. Dad, in particular, didn't trust "headshrinkers." But he couldn't help liking Bill and his wife, Laurel, who caused a stir in the community because they let their children run around naked. On our street of look-alike tract homes framed with nicely mowed lawns, the neighbors did not take to the Bastendorfs' jungle or their walls filled with posters of works by Picasso and Braque and Miró too. Sometimes Laurel would drive Mom to the only beatnik café in Santa Ana. Once there, they drank espresso coffee and talked about the latest *Sunset* magazine article on trendsetters like Charles Eames or Cliff May—something like that. All I know is, Mom ate it up, especially when Laurel showed her how to make shellboards. She was so inspired, she created her own hybrid—the Rockboard. Soon they were all over our house. The one I remember most was at least three by five feet and weighed so much that some of the rocks started to fall off.

Even though most people saw Dorothy as a housewife, I saw an artist struggling to find a medium.

Inspired by the Bastendorfs' example, in 1961 Mom piled us kids into the family station wagon and drove all the way to New York City to see the Art of Assemblage exhibition at the Museum of Modern Art. We were bowled over by Joseph Cornell and how he navigated an imaginary world through his boxes and collages. As soon as we got home, I decided to collage my entire bedroom wall. Mom was way into it, adding pictures from magazines she thought I might like, such as James Dean standing in Times Square. Soon she was collaging almost anything, including collage trash cans and collage storage boxes made with lumpy papier-mâché; she even collaged the inside of all the kitchen cabinets. (Don't ask.) Randy took it to a new level by becoming an actual collage artist. Even today, literally hundreds of his current series, "Stymied by a Woman's Face," are stacked in the oven, where he claims they're safe. I guess you could say collecting and reworking images, reorganizing the familiar into unexpected patterns in hopes of discovering something new, became one of our shared beliefs. Collage, like abstract reasoning, was a visual process for analyzing information. "Right?" as I always asked Mom when I was young. For sure she thought I was right.

I was fourteen when I started lugging around a memory I'll never let go. Mom and Dad were dancing in the moonlight on a hill in Ensenada, Mexico. A mariachi band played. I watched from the sidelines, as they kissed with a depth of feeling that should have been embarrassing for a teenage daughter. Instead, it filled me with awe. It even gave me something else to believe in. Their love. By lodging myself in the arms of Mother and Father's romance, I knew there would be no goodbyes.

On the last page of my teenage diary, I wrote: "To whom it may concern. When I get married I want my husband and I to talk serious matters over together. No emotional breakdowns in front of the kids. No swearing. I don't want my husband to smoke, but he can enjoy a good drink now and then. I want my children to go to Sunday school every Sunday. They will also get spankings, since I believe in them. In fact, I want my husband and I to run the household the same way Mom and Dad do right now."

"To whom it may concern"? Who was I kidding? And why was I trying to be such a good girl when what I really felt had nothing to do with pretend rules on a subject I was terrified of? This is what I didn't write down but have never forgotten. Dave Garland and I were passing notes in Mrs. Hopkins's ninth-grade algebra class one day. Dave was "really neat," but he "couldn't stand me." He ended our exchange with six words: "You'll make a good wife someday." A wife? I didn't want to be a wife. I wanted to be a hot date, someone to make out with. I wanted to be Barbra Streisand singing, "Never, never will I marry; born to wander till I'm dead." I never did marry. I never "went steady" either. While I dutifully continued to please my parents, my head was in the clouds, kissing unattainable greats like Dave Garland. I figured the only way to realize my number-one dream of be-

coming an actual Broadway musical comedy star was to remain an adoring daughter. Loving a man, and becoming a
wife, would have to be put aside. So I continued to pursue
unattainable greats.

The names changed, from Dave to Woody, then Warren,
and finally Al. Could I have made a lasting commitment to
them? Hard to say. Subconsciously I must have known it
could never work, and because of this they'd never get in the
way of my achieving my dreams. You see, I was looking for
bigger fish to fry. I was looking for an audience. Any audience. So what did I do? I auditioned for everything available
while mastering nothing in particular. I was in the church
choir and the school chorus. I tried out for cheerleader and
pom-pom girl. I auditioned for every talent show and every
play, including *The Taming of the Shrew*, which I didn't understand. I was a class debater and editor of the YWCA's
newsletter. I ran for ninth-grade secretary. I even begged
Mom to please help get me into Job's Daughters, a Masonic-
sponsored secret club where girls in a pageantlike atmosphere paraded around in long gowns. I wanted to be adored,
so I chose to stay safe in the arms of Jack and Dorothy; at
least, that's what I thought.

Now that I'm in my sixties, I want to understand more about
what it felt like to be the beautiful wife of Jack Hall, raising
four children in sunny California. I want to know why
Mother continually forgot to remember how wonderful she
was. I wish she would have taken pride in how much fun it
was for us to hear her play "My Mammy" on the piano and

sing, "The sun shines east, the sun shines west, I know where the sun shines best—Mammy." I don't know why she didn't appreciate how unusual it was when she took me to a room in a museum where a marble lion was missing the right side of his face; he also had no feet. The towering goddess in the other room had no arms. Mom was oohing and aahing, "Diane, isn't it beautiful?"

"But everything's lost. They don't have their parts," I said.

"But don't you see? Even without all their parts, look how magnificent they are." She was teaching me how to see. Yet she never took credit for anything. I wonder if her lack of self-esteem was an early symptom of forgetting. Was it really Alzheimer's that stole her memory, or was it a crippling sense of insecurity?

For fifteen years Mother kept saying goodbye: goodbye to names of places; goodbye to her famous tuna casseroles; goodbye to the BMW Dad bought her on her sixty-first birthday; goodbye to recognizing me as her daughter. Hello to Purina cat food molding on paper plates in her medicine chest; hello to caregivers; hello to the wheelchair guiding her to her favorite show—*Barney*—every morning on PBS; hello to the blank stare. Somewhere in the middle of the horrible hellos and tragic goodbyes, I adopted a baby girl. I was fifty. After a lifetime of avoiding intimacy, suddenly I got intimate in a big way. As Mother struggled to complete sentences, I watched Dexter, my daughter, and a few years later little Duke, my son, begin to form words as a means to capture the wonder of their developing minds.

The state of being a woman in between two loves—one

as a daughter, the other as a mother—has changed me. It's been a challenge to witness the betrayal of such a cruel disease while learning to give love with the promise of stability. If my mother was the most important person to me, if I am who and how I am largely due to who and how she was, what then does that say about my impact on Duke and Dexter? Abstract reasoning is no help.

At the beginning of her last year, Dorothy's small circle of devoted friends had all but fallen away. The people who loved her could be counted on one hand. It was hard to recognize the woman we had known. But then, am I recognizable as the same person I was when *Annie Hall* opened almost thirty-five years ago? I remember people coming up to me on the street, saying, "Don't ever change. Just don't ever change." Even Mom once said, "Don't grow old, Diane." I didn't like those words then, and I don't like them now. The exhausting effort to control time by altering the effects of age doesn't bring happiness. There's a word for you: *happiness*. Why is happiness something I thought I was entitled to? What is happiness anyway? *Insensitivity*. That's what Tennessee Williams said.

Mom's last word was *no*. No to the endless prodding. No to the unasked-for invasions. No to "Dinner, Dorothy?" "Time for your pills. Open your mouth." "We're going to roll you over, Mamacita." "NO!" "There, doesn't that feel good?" "NO!!" "Do you want to watch TV? *Lucy*'s on." "Let me get you a straw. Let me get you a fork." "NO." "Let me rub your shoulders." "No, no, no, no, NO!!!!" If she could, Mom would have said, "Leave me and my body alone, for God's sake. Don't touch me. This is my life. This is my ending." It wasn't that the activities were administered without affection and care; that wasn't the issue. The issue was independence. When I was a kid Mom would retreat to any unoccupied room with a longing that overshadowed her all-encompassing love for us. Once there, she would put aside the role of devoted mother, loving wife, and take refuge in her thoughts. In the end, *no* was all that was left of Dorothy's desire to have her wishes respected.

"Finally freed from the constraints of this life, Mom has joined Dad—just as she has joined her sisters, Orpha and Martha; her mother, Beulah; and all her dear cats, starting with Charcoal, ending with Cyrus. I promise to take care of her thoughts and words. I promise to THINK. And I promise to carry the legacy of beautiful, beautiful Dorothy Deanne Keaton Hall from Kansas, born on October thirty-first, 1921—my mother."

I spoke these words at her memorial service in November 2008. Mom continues to be the most important, influential person in my life. From the outside looking in, we lived completely different lives. She was a housewife and mother who dreamed of success; I am an actress whose life has been—in some respects—beyond my wildest dreams. Comparing two women with big dreams who shared many of the same conflicts and also happened to be mother and daughter is partially a story of what's lost in success contrasted with what's gained in accepting an ordinary life. I was an ordinary girl who became an ordinary woman, with one exception: Mother gave me extraordinary will. It didn't come free. But, then, life wasn't a free ride for Mother either.

So why did I write a memoir? Because Mom lingers; because she tried to save our family's history through her words; because it took decades before I recognized that her most alluring trait was her complexity; because I don't want her to disappear even though she has. So many reasons, but the best answer comes from a passage she wrote using those fine abstract-reasoning capabilities she passed on to me. The year was 1980. She was fifty-nine.

Every living person should be forced to write an autobiography. They should have to go back and unravel and disclose all the stuff that was packed into their lives. Finding the unusual way authors put ideas into words gives me a very satisfying knowledge that I could do this too if I focused on it. It might help me release the pressure I feel from stored up memories that are affecting me now. But I do something terribly wrong. I tell myself I'm too controlled by my past habits. I really want to write about my life, the close friends I knew, the family life we had, but I hold back. If I would be totally honest, I think I could reach a point where I'd begin seeing ME in a more understandable light. Now I'm jumpy in my recollected thought, yet I know it would be nothing but good for me to do this.

I wish she had. And, because she didn't, I've written not my memoir but ours. The story of a girl whose wishes came true because of her mother is not new, but it's mine. The profound love and gratitude I feel now that she's left has compelled me to try to "unravel" the mystery of her journey.

In so doing I hoped to find the meaning of our relationship and understand why realized dreams are such a strange burden. What I've done is create a book that combines my own memories and stories with Mom's notebooks and journals. Thinking back to her scrapbooks and our mutual love of collage, I've placed her words beside mine, along with letters, clippings, and other materials that document not just our lives but our bond. I want to hold my life up alongside hers in order to, as she wrote, reach a point where I begin to see *me*—and *her*—in a more understandable light.

PART ONE

1

DOROTHY

Extraordinary

Dorothy's commitment to writing began with a letter to Ensign Jack Hall, who was stationed with the Navy in Boston. It was just after the end of World War II. She was resting in the Queen of Angels Hospital after having given birth to me. All alone with a seven-pound, seven-ounce baby, she began a correspondence that would develop into a different kind of passion. At that time, Mom's words were influenced by the few movies Beulah had allowed her to see, like 1938's *Broadway Melody*. Harmless fluff pieces with dialogue out of the mouth of Judy Garland. Mom's "I sure do love you more than anything in the world" and her use of "swell" and "No one could ever make me happier than you" mirrored the American worldview of life and its expectations during the

1940s. For Dorothy, more than anything, it was love. It was Jack. It was Diane, and it was swell.

Mom wrote her first "Hello, Honey" letter when I was eight days old. Fifty years later I met my daughter, Dexter, and held her in my arms when she was eight days old. She was a cheerful baby. Contrary to my long-held belief, I was not a cheerful baby or even very cute. Mother's concern about my appearance was defined by a bad photograph. Photography was already telling people how to see me. I didn't pass Dad's pretty-picture test, or Mom's for that matter. Holed up in Grammy Keaton's little bungalow on Monterey Road in Highland Park, Dorothy had no choice. Through her twenty-four-year-old eyes she wanted to believe I was extraordinary. I had to be. She passed this kind of hope on to a baby girl who got caught up in its force. Our six months alone together sealed the deal. Everything for Dorothy became heightened because she was exploding with the joy, pain, fear, and empathy of being a first-time mother.

January 13, 1946
Dearest Jack,

You should be just about getting into Boston, and I'll bet you are pretty worn out from the trip. It's hard to realize it could be so cold there when it's so nice here. I'm sorry I acted the way I did when you left. I sure didn't want to, but the thought of you leaving got me so upset. I tried awfully hard to stop crying, because I knew it wasn't good for Diane.

It's 8:00 p.m., and your daughter's asleep. She's getting prettier every day and by the time you see

*her you may decide to have her for your "favorite
dish." That's not fair, honey—I saw you first, so I
should be first choice in your harem, don't you think?
Chiquita and Lois came over today. They agreed she
was swell, even though she has one bad habit—
whenever anyone comes to look at her she looks back
at them cross-eyed.*

*Well, honey, I think I'll wake little "Angel Face" up.
We've certainly got a prize, no fooling. Every time I look
at her I think I can't wait until you can see her, and we
can be by ourselves.*
Good night, my love,
Dorothy

January 18, 1946
Hello, Honey,
*I wish I wasn't such a crybaby. I don't understand
me. Until I was married you couldn't make me cry over
anything. I thought I couldn't cry—but now all I have
to do is think of you and how swell you are and I miss
you so much before I know it I'm bawling just like
Diane. I sure do love you more than you could know,
honey. Even if I don't tell you very often when I see
you, I'm always thinking it.*

*Diane & I had our picture taken—just small cheap
ones. I'm afraid they can't be too good of her—she's so
tiny—and naturally they won't be good of me, but
that's to be expected. I hope you can at least see what
she looks like a little bit. The photographer said she was
very good for a baby her size & age. She's not fat like*

her mother used to be. *Incidentally I'm still on the plump side = darn it. She weighs over 9 lbs. and, as I say in every letter—gets cuter everyday. I think that's a nice idea of yours, sending her $2.00 bills. I'm putting them away for her. It's adding up. Maybe pretty soon we could start a savings account for her. Good night, my Honey.*
Love,
Dorothy

February 21, 1946
Hello, Honey,

I'm so disappointed. Those pictures are just as I expected—awful. Diane looks kind of funny. I'm not going to send them cause you'll think I've been kidding you about how cute she is.

You said in your letter today that you wish we could relive those good old days again. I sure look back and dream about how swell they were. We don't want to ever change, do we? Even though we have a family and more responsibilities, I don't think that's any reason to act older and not have the fun we used to. Right?!
Good night, Darling Jack,
Your Dorothy

March 31, 1946
Dear Jack,

Right now I'm so mad at you I could really tell you off if you were here. I don't know whatever gave you *the crazy idea that I might have changed and "start liking someone else." You aren't the only person that believes in making a success of their marriage—it means just as much to me as it does you, and if you think I go around looking for someone that might suit me a little better, you don't think too much of me. Don't you think I take being married seriously? You ought to know how much I love you—so why in the world would I try and find someone else? You said you wanted me to be happy—well, believe me, you couldn't make me any more unhappy if you tried. If you would just have a little confidence in me and trust me more you wouldn't think such things. You don't have to keep reminding me of the fact that we promised to tell each other first if things had changed. That applies to you too. Would you like it if I kept telling you I didn't think it would last long and you would soon find someone else? Well, I sure don't like it one bit so please don't write like that again.*

I probably shouldn't send this but the more I think about it the madder I get! But no matter how mad I get, honey—I love you as much as I can and if I looked the whole world over I couldn't see anyone but you because no one could ever make me any happier than you always have and always will. I feel better now—not mad anymore, but I'll be really mad if you ever write that way again—don't forget.

Love,

Dorothy

P.S. I've decided to send you our photographs after all.

April 25, 1946

Hello, Honey,

   *So you didn't like the pictures, huh? Please don't
think your daughter looks like that because I assure you
she doesn't. And even if she wasn't cute, she would be
darling just from her personality alone. She has one
already—very definitely. I think I'll wait awhile before I
have her picture taken again.*

   *You know, of course, that we have a very
remarkable and intelligent daughter. I was reading my
baby book about what a 4-month-old baby should be
doing and she was doing everything they mentioned
when she was 2 months, really. She tries her hardest to
sit up, and they don't do that until they are 5 or 6
months. She really does take after you in every way—
looks, smartness, and personality. Don't worry, she will
surely be a beauty.*

   *Well, honey, only 38 more days until that wonderful
day when I see you again. Diane said, "Whoopee!"
Well, anyway, she smiled—*

Bye, honey,

Love,

Dorothy

Looking West

My first memory is of shadows creating patterns on a wall.
Inside my crib, I saw the silhouette of a woman with long
hair move across the bars. Even as she picked me up and held

me, my mother was a mystery. It was almost as if I knew the world, and life in it, would be unfamiliar yet charged with an alluring, permanent, and questioning romance. As if I would spend the rest of my life trying to understand her. Is this memory real? I don't know.

Certain things stand out: the snowstorm in Los Angeles when I was three; the Quonset hut we lived in until I was five. It had a wonderful shape. I've loved arches ever since. One night, Mr. Eigner, our next-door neighbor, caught me singing "Over the Rainbow" on Daddy's newly paved driveway. I thought I was going to get into trouble. Instead, he told me I was a "mighty talented young lady." Daddy worked at the Department of Water and Power in downtown Los Angeles. I'd go visit him at his office when I was five. There was something about looking west from the Angels Flight trolley car that mesmerized me. Tall buildings like City Hall peeked over the hill. I loved Clifton's Cafeteria and the Broadway department store. Everything was condensed and concrete and angled and bustling with activity. Downtown was perfect. I thought heaven must look like Los Angeles. But nothing compared to the joy of tugging on Mom's arm, telling her to "Look! Look, Mom." We both loved looking.

It was hard to know what Mom loved more, looking or writing. Her scrapbooks, at least when I was a little girl, were ruined by endless explanations underneath the photographs. As I got older, I avoided the unwanted envelopes with her "Letters to Diane" like the plague. Who cared about letters? I just wanted pictures. After my incident in the darkroom with Mother's journal, that was it for me. But when I made the decision to write a memoir at age sixty-three, I

began to read Mother's journals in no particular order. In
the middle of this process, I came across what must have
been an attempt at her own memoir. Embossed in gold at the
top of the cover was *1980*. That meant she began to write it
when she was fifty-nine. Each entry was dated. Sometimes
Mom would start an excerpt, then stop, leaving dozens of
pages empty. Or she would write a paragraph on an incident
one year, only to return to it a couple of years later, only to
restart with yet another approach months after. Over the
course of five years, she skipped in and out of her childhood
events almost as if she was free-associating. For the most
part Dorothy's tone was forgiving, sweet, and sometimes ele-
giac. But sometimes it wasn't. She must have been taking
stock of her life by dredging up memories of those days in
the thirties when she was sandwiched between the harsh
rules laid down by the Free Methodist church and the lure of
life outside Beulah's constraints. I hate to believe it's true,
but life threw Dorothy some punches she didn't recover
from.

Family Feelings

*My father, Roy Keaton, nicknamed me Perkins when I was
very young, maybe three or four years old. He used it when
he had "family feelings." When he felt estranged, he called
me Dorothy. Daddy made it clear with all three of Mother's
pregnancies that he wanted a boy. As we girls grew, it became obvious that I was the one he wished had been the
boy of his dreams. I was the tomboy, a quiet girl who gave*

no one trouble. I don't know why Dad favored me over my
sisters. Sometimes he confided thoughts he didn't even
share with Mother. I always listened wordlessly. When he
finished he would say, "Isn't that right, Perkins, huh? Huh?"
He knew I would always agree. I think he also knew I always agreed with Mother too.

We moved a lot. When I was 4 we lived in an old
two-story frame house on Walnut St. in Pasadena. The
house sat right on the sidewalk. But we had a huge yard
that backed up to the railroad tracks, which carried the new
Super Chief Santa Fe train. No fence, or wall, or anything
separated our yard from the track. I saw passengers' faces
as they looked into our kitchen. Today this would not be
permissible but no one cared back then. Dad's German
shepherd, Grumpy, would sleep on the tracks, but he always ambled off just in time.

We always had cats. I was still just a kid when we
moved to a cheaper rental house on top of a hill in Highland Park. It was set on a half acre of loose dirt, with a
small patch of grass. We didn't have neighbors. Very few
people cared to climb the steep public stairway from the
street. It was a perfect setting for cats. Mom let me have all
I wanted. 13. Dad couldn't have cared less. He was seldom
there anyway. Money was scarce. Somehow these little
furry creatures got fed every day along with the five of us. I
found Pretty Boy, Cakes, Yeller, and Alex in one week. One
particular cat though dominates my memory. Her name
was Baby. She was a dull gray thing, with skinny legs, and
eyes that made up most of her head, and a broken tail that
hung crooked. The strangest thing was she made no sounds;

*no meows; no hisses and no purrs. Baby was a genetic fail-
ure to everyone but me. I loved her. One day, she gave birth
to a litter of four kittens. To my great sorrow, though, Baby
was never the same. She died not long after. Orpha didn't
care that much. She already had boyfriends she didn't tell
Mother about, so she was constantly sneaking out in the
middle of the night. Marti was just a little girl, so she
didn't pay attention to them, but to me, the cats were the
dearest things in the whole wide world. Mother always said
being the middle sister made me the most sensitive. I don't
know about that, but it made me sad we couldn't share
how special they were. I never told them about my dream
of owning a big cat farm where I could save every orphan
cat I ever saw, broken down or not.*

Firstborn

Being firstborn had its advantages. I had Mom and Dad all
to myself. Then Randy arrived, my junior by a couple of
years. Randy was sensitive—too sensitive. As president and
creator of the Beaver Club, I made Randy, the treasurer,
come with me to the public stairway near the arroyo to look
for money. Our number-one mission was to buy coonskin
caps like Davy Crockett's. They cost a dollar and ninety-eight
cents apiece. We were beside ourselves when Randy spotted
an actual honest-to-God fifty-cent piece. Wow. Since I was
president of the Beaver Club, it was my self-appointed responsibility to handle all finances, so I picked it up and held
it in my hand for one perfect instant before Randy started

screaming. I looked up and saw an airplane gliding across the sky in slow motion. Big deal. But Randy was so terrified I couldn't stop him from running home in tears and hiding under our bunk bed. Even Mom couldn't convince him it was only an airplane. After that, Randy became seriously hesitant about the outside world, especially about flying objects. In his teens it was almost impossible to pry him out of his room down the hall. Robin was convinced he was disappearing, and he was: He was disappearing into Frank Zappa, whose lyrics to songs like "Zomby Woof" became his mantra.

Mom and Dad worried about him right from the get-go. I made use of their concern by willing myself to be everything Randy wasn't. Big mistake. What I didn't understand was that his sensitivity allowed him to perceive the world with intensity and insight.

It was almost too easy to manipulate him out of items like his one and only green Duncan Tournament Yo-Yo, or the Big Hunk candy bar he saved from Halloween, or one of his very special cat's-eye marbles he hid under the bunk bed. Sure, he was more unique and intuitive, but what did I care as long as I got what I wanted?

When Robin came along three years after Randy, I was beside myself with envy. A girl? How was that possible? Surely there was some mistake. She must have been adopted. Of course, she turned out pretty and she had a better singing voice than I did, but, worse than all that, she was Daddy's favorite. Many years later, it drove me nuts when Warren Beatty referred to Robin as the "pretty, sexy sister."

Dorrie came as an "unexpected surprise." I was seven

years older, so she could do no wrong. Her face was a minia-
ture replica of Dorothy's. She was the brightest, most intel-
lectually gifted of the Hall kids. In fact, she was the only one
of us who ever presented Mom and Dad with a report card
of straight A's. She loved to read biographies of inspirational
women like Simone de Beauvoir and Anaïs Nin. She read *A
Spy in the House of Love* because it was a good "message"
book. She said it instilled in her an optimistic outlook toward
the future. She thought I might find some tidbits to apply to
my philosophy on "love." I didn't have a philosophy on love.
That's what hooked me on Dorrie; she was full of contradictions. It must have been part of the terms of being our only
"intellectual."

We spent all weekends and every vacation at the sea-
shore. In 1955, Huntington Beach still gave permission for
families to pitch tents on the water's edge for a month at a
time. Ours rose out of the sand like a black cube. That was
the summer I read *The Wonderful Wizard of Oz* and *The
Adventures of Perrine*. I was nine. It seemed like life would
always be imbued with black words on white pages, framed
by white waves and black nights. Mom put zinc oxide on my
nose every morning before Randy and I collected pop bottles, stacked them into borrowed shopping carts, and depos-
ited them at the A&P supermarket for two cents apiece.
With money in our pockets, we were able to buy our way into
the famous heated saltwater swimming pool. A few years
later, Dad took us farther south and assembled our tent at
Doheny Beach, where we caught waves on six-foot Hobie
surfboards and sang songs like "Hang Down Your Head,
Tom Dooley" around the campfire. Sometimes we'd drive up

to Rincon, where we set up camp at the side of the Pacific
Coast Highway. But it was Divers Cove in Laguna Beach that
had Daddy's heart. He and his best friend, Bob Blandin,
would slip into their wet suits and disappear under the
ocean's surface for hours at a time while we kids played on
the shore. Mom packed bologna sandwiches with mayon-
naise. Willie, Bob's wife, wore Chinese red lipstick and
smoked, which Mom said was *really bad*. I remember the
cliffs. At night they looked like dinosaurs ready to attack us.
During the day we climbed them to the top and looked out
over our beloved Laguna Beach. If you had seen us from the
beach below, you would've thought we were the picture-
perfect average California family in the fifties.

One Man's Family

*The radio played a big part in our life. The one I remember
most was a tall cabinet model made by Philco. We bought it
on time, as we did with everything of value. Sundays were
Radio Day. One Man's Family was on at 3. It was my favorite. My sisters and I hurried home from church in order
to follow the plot of Father Barber and his perfectly neat
family. There just couldn't be anyone as good, or wise, or
understanding as Father Barber. I thought it unfair that I
couldn't have a father who would give big hugs and talk
and laugh with his daughter. I always wondered how come
my dad wasn't like that, all warm and patient and loving
and . . . well, he just wasn't, that's all!! "If only" he would
just say, "Come over here, Perkins, and give your dad a*

kiss." If only Mom would say, "Hurry up, I know how exciting the next episode of the Barber family is for you."

The only thing our family had in common with the serials was Mom and Dad were always looking for a better life. I thought it was unfair. And when I grew up I wasn't going to live the way we did. My family would be perfect. I would see to that; always and forever happy, smiling, and beautiful.

Unanswered Questions

When I was six, television gave me a gift. Gale Storm. Not Lucille Ball. Gale Storm in *My Little Margie*. She was everything I wanted to be—clever, fearless, and always up to wacky antics that invariably got her into big trouble with her father. She was funny but fragile. I liked that. *I Love Lucy* was television's number-one highest-rated sitcom. Gale Storm's knockoff was number two, but not to me. Gale and I were kindred spirits, or so I thought. After 126 episodes, *My Little Margie* was canceled. It was a sad day.

Fifteen years later, when I was a student at the Neighborhood Playhouse School of the Theatre, Phil Bonnell, the son of Gale Storm, was one of my classmates. On Christmas break he invited me to his mother's home in Beverly Hills. This is what I remember. It was noon. Gale Storm was nowhere to be found. Phil told me she slept late. I thought everyone's mother was up at six A.M. with hot Cream of Wheat and the voice of Bob Crane, the King of the Los Angeles Airwaves, blaring on the radio. There was no radio playing at the Bonnells' house, an uncomfortable, rambling ranch-style affair. When Gale finally came out, she wasn't lively, and there were no antics. Later, Phil told me she drank a lot. Gale Storm drank? That's when it dawned on me: Everything wasn't perfect for Gale Storm, even though it seemed her dreams had come true.

I found my next hero in high school: Gregory Peck. Well, Gregory Peck as Atticus Finch in *To Kill a Mockingbird*. His unassuming, quiet approach to solving the moral dilemmas of life inspired me. My worship for him was even greater than my teen crush on Warren Beatty in *Splendor in the Grass*.

I always told Mom everything—well, everything except my feelings about intercourse and movie stars like Warren Beatty. Gregory Peck, however, was discussed over and over. If only there was a way to meet him. Mom had to understand how he alone could teach me to be the kind of person I wanted to be, a hero in my own right. Under his guidance, I would have the courage to rescue people from the injustice of a racist community or even put my life on the line for what I believed.

Always encouraging, Mom let me roam through some pretty undeveloped thoughts. One time I told her about how frustrating Dad was. According to him, I never did anything right. He was always saying, "Don't sit too close to the TV or you'll go blind," or "Finish the food on your plate; there's starving people in China," and, my least favorite, "Don't chew with your mouth open unless you want to catch flies." Was there something about being a civil engineer that made him that way? Was that the reason he never thought I did things right? Mom was different. She didn't judge me or try to tell me what to think. She let me think.

Grandfather Keaton

*The word came late one February night. It was a
long-distance phone call from Oklahoma. An emergency.
Had to be. There was no other reason for calling in 1937.
Daddy took the call. "Come get your father. We can't keep
him any longer."*

*Dad couldn't possibly leave work, so it was decided
that Mother and I would bring Grandpa to live out his days
with us. I would unfortunately have to miss two weeks of
school. I pretended "answering the call of an emergency"
was a duty I was obliged to fulfill. Secretly I was thrilled.*

*We set out with 25 dollars in cash, two gas credit cards,
our California clothes, and a 1936 Buick Sedan. We took
Route 66 through Kingman, Flagstaff, and Gallup on
through to Oklahoma. When we arrived at our relatives'
home, Grandpa was ready. All his worldly possessions were
in a small worn suitcase. His hair was unkempt, but he
smiled at us with tears in his eyes. We were told he was incapable of expressing a thought.*

*Grandfather Keaton had been a lazy if good-hearted
man. Roy's mother, Anna, bore the burden. Eventually she
had to go to work. When she insisted the marriage end, un-
heard of in those days, Grandpa began roaming the country
in a red Model T Ford truck accompanied by his dog
"Buddy." Over time things deteriorated, and Grandpa came
back home. Anna took him in until she became so frustrated she called us in the dead of winter to come take him
away.*

On our trip back home, Grandpa seemed happy. He no sooner stepped into the backseat of the Buick before he leaned forward and handed Mother a huge wad of bills. Our trip home was full of many more comforts than the trip going, but we paid for it. Dressing Grandpa in the morning was impossible. He put his pants on backwards. He couldn't get his arms in his jacket. He didn't know how to tie his shoes. He refused to wear socks. He didn't have any table manners, or teeth, for that matter. His baggy trousers were damp all the time. He was incontinent. This annoyed Mother to no end. We put in long, long hours driving in order to make it back in three and a half days.

Needless to say it was a whole new life with Grandpa occupying one of our 3 bedrooms. Dad refused to participate in his father's care at all. That was Mother's job. The details were unbelievable. Grandpa would sneak out of the house and run away at least twice a week. Mother had to go looking for him all over the neighborhood. Finally, we locked him in his room. He would pound on the door so loud he caused the neighbors to complain. When his bowels became impacted, Mom forced Dad to give him an enema. The results were so awful the toilet plugged up. It didn't take long for us to decide that Grandpa's condition was beyond home care. Arrangements were made to transfer him to the veterans hospital on Sawtelle in Los Angeles. Dad drug his feet on this, but Mother insisted.

The last time I saw Grandpa he was waving goodbye from a car driving him to the old soldiers' section of the veterans hospital. Dad never forgave Mother, even though he never bothered to lift a finger to help. I'm ashamed to say, Martha and I gave Mother no help either. We were teenage girls, and Grandpa was an embarrassment. Later I found out that while Mom was burdened with the hardship of caring for Grandpa, Dad was seeing another woman. It wasn't long after this he drove off, never to return.

The Sea of White Crosses

Five days a week for the past four years, I've taken a shortcut through the very same veterans hospital off San Vicente near Sawtelle. On the north side of the complex is the graveyard Duke refers to as "the Sea of White Crosses." Sometimes I tell him about all the soldiers who lived and died to help keep our country safe. He always wants to know if they looked like the green plastic soldiers we buy at Target.

Until I read Mother's words, I didn't know the story of an incontinent, wandering Keaton fellow who shared a house with his young granddaughter Dorothy, who was on the eve of meeting a certain Jack Newton Hall, who would become my father. How is it possible that I could have driven by Duke's Sea of White Crosses for so many years without knowing my great-grandfather Lemuel W. Keaton Jr.'s cross was so close to home?

Sermons

All sermons were always about the resurrection of the living Christ Jesus of Nazareth, born to save mankind from

*the threat of an eternity in Hell. The catch was you had to
be born again. I played it safe. I read my Bible and pro-
claimed in testimony at prayer meetings that I indeed was
saved, sanctified, and born again. Whenever I had the courage to stand up and state my memorized passage, the entire
congregation smiled. I never understood what my declara-
tion meant. I just wanted church to be colorful. I just
wanted beautiful music like Handel's* Messiah *and Cop-
land's* Appalachian Spring. *I didn't want to hear about
Blood and Death. Yet this was the ritual you couldn't avoid.
Blood. Sin. Guilt. Tears. Death. Shroud. Tomb. It was nothing more than a relinquishing of our free will to a philosophy that all men are born in sin and must be forgiven and
saved from themselves in order to qualify for eternal and
everlasting peace. It has taken all my 60 years to straighten
out my thinking on all this, and believe me I am finally un-
burdened. I am free of the fear instilled in me, free from the
angry God, the straight and narrow path to Heaven, and
the fiery anguish of living in Hell. I am grateful to whatever
force in the universe there is that has removed me of all the
ugliness imposed on me by false ideas about what life
should be. And when I'm through with my time in the
scheme of it all, I'm not afraid of what comes after. Amen.*

Playing with Death

When I was ten we moved to Garden Grove for six months.
Dad rented a house with a rock roof. The man and woman
who owned it were brassy. She had bleached-blond hair, and

he owned a bar. Dad called them "alcoholics." I'd never heard that word before. It meant they drank a lot of liquor. Dad said the landlords were slobs. He was right. The house was a mess, but it had four bedrooms and two baths. It was the biggest house I'd ever seen, way bigger than the blue stucco house he had moved in a truck to Bushnell Way Road in Highland Park. The kitchen had swinging doors, like the ones in *Gunsmoke*, starring James Arness. Dorrie and Robin shared a bedroom. Randy, who was eight, had his own room, like me.

One day Robin was playing with friends in the backyard. I wanted to join in, but nobody cared, especially Robin. I decided to take one of the ropes from our swing set, wrap it around my neck, and pretend I was hanging myself. When Robin ran past me without so much as a nod, I started to make loud choking sounds. Surely that would make her come to her senses. But, oh no, she kept on playing. So I showed her. I slumped my head over the rope even farther, gagged as loudly as I could, took a deep breath, let out a scream, and died. She never noticed.

With my face knotted up in tears, I ran inside and told Mom that Robin let me die. She looked at me and asked why did it matter so much whether they played with me or not? Death, even a pretend death, was not the way to get what I wanted. It was not a game. In her face I saw what I hadn't seen in Robin's. Concern. The truth is, I would have done the whole stupid thing over again just to have her wrap her arms around me so tight I could feel her heart beat.

Mom's empathy was bottomless, an endless source of renewal. I can still see her sipping her afternoon cup of Folgers coffee while I sat across the kitchen counter in some form of distress. It was a scene we would relive in endless variations throughout the years. Her message was always the same. "Don't be so sensitive, Diane. You'll show them one day. Go for it." And, like clockwork, even if I failed I kept going for it, not only because I longed for validation but also because I wanted to come back to her and that kitchen counter for as long as forever would last.

Those days were terribly puzzling, especially when I became aware that Robin had no interest in playing the part I wrote for her or that alcoholics drank stuff that made them bad people, much worse than Willie Blandin and her bad cigarettes. But the worst, most bewildering, awful thing came the day Daddy took it upon himself to tell me I was about to become a woman soon. A woman? Was he crazy? I ran to my bedroom, slammed the door, and threw myself on the bed facedown. Mom came in a little later and said I was going to love being a grown-up girl. I didn't want to hurt her feelings, but I was disgusted. I didn't want a period, whatever that was, or breasts, or hair in my privacy area, like her. I didn't want to be a woman. I wanted to be me—whoever that was.

Bloody Sunday

Easter Sunday was as important and exciting as Christmas. The beauty of the day, so big in the world of Christianity, was never given much play. Instead, we were told in long-winded sermons about the cruel crucifixion of Jesus

Christ, our savior who died on the cross, shedding his blood to save us . . . ME. I could never grasp the meaning of this idea. Our hymns were burdened with words like: "Washed in the Blood of the lamb." "I'm saved by the Blood of Christ." "He shed his precious Blood for me." Blood, the big symbol, meant absolutely nothing to me.

Easter meant one thing, a complete new outfit. Mother would begin making my dress early. My favorite was a pink ankle-length gown with a deep ruffle on the bottom and at the neck. We all bought new shoes and new hats. All the ladies and young girls in their springtime finery would parade around the grounds of the old Free Methodist church. It was our version of the Easter Parade. I loved it.

Save It for Later

Even before I was a teenager, I realized something was wrong. Being the first of four children, I couldn't understand why all the attractive genes had been passed on to my younger sisters, Robin and Dorrie. This incredible botch job had to be corrected. I hated my nose, so I slept with a bobby pin stuck on top, hoping the bulb would squeeze into a straight line. In Mom's bathroom mirror I spent hours practicing a special smile, convinced it would hide my flaws. I even pried my eyes open as wide as possible for hours, determined they'd grow bigger.

A few years later, my best friend, Leslie Morgan, and I slunk through the hallways of Santa Ana High School like dark smudges in a universe of red, white, and blue. Unrecognizable in our white lipstick and black eyeliner, we tried to be pretty by renouncing normalcy. At the beginning of every month, we'd sneak over to Sav-on drugstore in Honer Plaza to see if the new *Vogue* was out. We loved Penelope Tree; her bangs were so long they almost covered her face. I decided to cut bangs too—long ones. They hid my forehead, but they didn't solve the problem. The problem was my fixation with pretty. Mom gave no guidance with regard to my face. Sometimes I thought she didn't have much hope for me in that department. But she had plenty of ideas about style. In fact, it might have been better if she had given me a little less freedom of expression in the fashion department.

But, hey, I thought we were a pretty good team. By the time I was fifteen, I designed most of my clothes and Mom sewed them. When I say *designed,* I mean I played around with the patterns we bought by changing details. The basic shape remained the same. Mom was a big proponent of the "walk-away" dress. It was so easy to make you could "start it after breakfast . . . walk away in it for lunch!" Fabric was essential. Everything available at Woolworth's or Penney's was entirely too predictable. Mom and I branched out and hit the Goodwill thrift shop, where we found a treasure trove of search-and-rescue items waiting for us in polka dots, stripes, and English plaids. We cut up men's old tweed jackets and made patchwork miniskirts. Of course, Mom carried the heavy load. I had no interest in learning how to sew. God, no. Results were all that mattered—quick results and The Look.

I was unaware that Mother had questions about my

"appearance" until I found something she wrote in 1962. Under the heading "Diane," she observed: *Diane's hair is ratted at least four inches high. Her skirts are three inches above the knees, and while we all kid her to death on this, the total effect is pretty cute, I guess. To us here at home, she looks her best at night, when all the rats are out and she is in her comfortable pants with no eye makeup. She is quite a girl, in this junior year of high school. She has an independent way about her. She shows a set of values she has figured out for herself. She is strong on this point. A sure way to lose an argument with Diane is to tell her what she should do or think. She has to decide for herself.*

And I did, thanks to her. My all-time favorite outfit was this little getup we put together for my high school graduation ceremony in 1963. After I redesigned the Simplicity pattern of a minidress Mom bought at Newberry's, where I worked in the ladies' bra department, we hit the Goodwill and found the perfect black-and-white polka-dot fabric from an old shirtwaist dress with a wide skirt. Then we splurged and bought an expensive pair of white straw high heels with pointed toes and black pom-poms. I found some black seamed stockings to go with it so I could look more mod. I even had a theory: If I hid my face, if I framed it to highlight my best feature, which I figured was my smile, I would get more attention. But then something happened that changed my life. I was browsing around our other favorite store, the Salvation Army thrift shop, when I found the answer: a hat, a man's old bowler hat. I put it on my head—and that was it!

For the first time, Mom put her foot down. "I love it, but not for this occasion, Diane."

When I showed up at graduation, I still achieved the effect I wanted. My smile stood out, and I got a lot of attention. It didn't matter if I looked ridiculous; I beat the odds of being plain old average Diane. And Mom was right about the hat. Better to save it for later.

2
JACK

Not in the Cards

When I was little, I didn't get my dad. He did nothing but remind me to turn off the lights, shut the refrigerator door, and eat what Mom cooked or I'd have to sleep in the garage. He wore the same gray jacket and striped tie to the Department of Water and Power every day. He said, "Drink all your milk; it gives you strong bones," "Be sure to say please and thank you," and, always, "Ask questions." Why was he like that? Over and over I would ask Mom. Over and over she would say he was busy and had a lot of important things on his mind. He had things on his mind? What were they? She didn't help me understand my father at all. The only clue lived a few miles away, but everyone was afraid of her, and I was no exception.

It wasn't Grammy Keaton; oh, no, it was all five feet ten

inches of stern-faced brown-haired Grammy Hall. She used to say she didn't cotton to dressing up in a lot of gay colors, 'cause she "occupied a lot of space" and wanted everybody to see her "plain." Grammy Keaton said the reason Dad had rickets was because Mrs. Hall hadn't fed him the kind of nutritious food that would have made his legs straight; instead, they bowed backward, like a sailboat. She wasn't wrong.

Even though Grammy Hall lived close to Grammy Keaton, they did not become friends. It was easy to see why. Grammy Hall's face was lined with skepticism, while Grammy Keaton's was filled with faith. Every Sunday, Grammy Keaton baked angel food cake with seven-minute frosting, served with homemade ice cream and lemonade in tall glasses. Once a year, Grammy Hall made devil's food cake from a mix. Grammy Keaton was a God-fearing Christian woman. Grammy Hall was a devout Catholic. Grammy Keaton believed in heaven. Grammy Hall thought it was "a lot of bunk."

After her husband disappeared in the 1920s, Mary Alice Hall drove from Nebraska to California with her son, Jack, and her sister Sadie beside her. It couldn't have been easy being a boy without a father in the twenties. Mary Hall offered no explanations. There's still some question whether Dad was a bastard or if in fact, as Mary claimed, Chester had died before Jack was born. Whatever the truth, Mary, a tough, no-nonsense Irish Catholic, picked herself up and waved goodbye to her eleven brothers and sisters, her mother, her father, and the broken-down family farm in Nebraska. She didn't look back.

Nobody knows where she got the money to buy a two-unit Spanish duplex just a few blocks north of the new 110 freeway, but she did. Mary leased out the bottom floor to her sister Sadie, Sadie's husband, Eddie, and their change-of-life son, Cousin Charlie. Mary shared the second floor with George Olsen, who rented the bedroom at the end of the hallway, next to Dad's room. It wasn't clear what George meant to Mary. No one asked. Grammy did not invite questions about her personal life.

Mary lived at 5223 Range View Avenue until she died in the dining room, the same dining room Mom and Dad dragged us to every Thanksgiving. One year I snuck down the hall, went into her bedroom, carefully opened her chest of drawers, and found a bunch of quarters shoved into several pairs of old socks. I was so excited I even told Cousin Charlie, who couldn't be bothered with me since we'd had a fight over his stupid Catholic God. He said I was an idiot and a bunch of quarters was chicken feed compared to the sacks of hundred-dollar bills he'd found stuffed under the floorboards in her coat closet.

Grammy was more man than woman, and looked it. She loved to describe herself as a self-made businesswoman who took in boarders. "What interests me is the world of commerce. I like to make a lot of money and make it quick." In fact, Mary Alice Hall was a loan shark, who shamelessly went around the neighborhood collecting currency at high interest rates from people who were down on their luck. She had one goal in life: the acquisition and retention of cash, lots of it. This "make no bones about it" attitude applied to her choice of a newspaper as well. She proudly subscribed to the *Herald Express*, "a paper aimed at the underside of the community, the kind of people who wanted to know about murders and UFOs and sports results." She wasn't highfalutin. She understood people who disappeared into the thin air of a lousy marriage, a failed bank account, or a petty crime. Why wouldn't she want to read about the plethora of commonplace sad stories that made up most people's lives?

Mary's idea of motherhood was simple: If Jack misbehaved, she locked him in the closet and walked away. Nothing more. Nothing less. When her good-for-nothing card-shark brother Emmet was down on his luck, she made little Jackie share a room with him. She must have figured, what the hell, she could use the extra money. According to Dad, Emmet was immoral. Right before Dad enrolled at USC, Emmet cheated him out of a hundred dollars. They didn't speak for two years, even though they continued to share the same room. Dad hated Emmet, but their forced alliance produced something positive. Jack Hall did not become a lying cheat like his stinky-cigar-smoking uncle.

Dad never knew his father's first name. As with everyone else, he didn't ask. Mary made sure no one mentioned a man called Chester. Aunt Sadie followed her marching orders and kept her mouth shut. Mom too. The last thing Dorothy wanted was a confrontation with her mother-in-law. Stirring it up with Mary Alice Hall was not worth it. The mystery remained unsolved until I discovered a newspaper article in Mom's file cabinet.

Wife Hunts 9 Years for Husband;
Asks for Insurance.

Monday June 23, 1930. Positive He's Dead,
She Declares; Husband Vanished Three Months
After Marriage.

Somewhat like Evangeline was Mrs. Mary Hall. Only she didn't stick it out as long as the girl of the romantic verse. She searched from coast to coast, seeking Chester N. Hall, who nine years ago left her, when she was his bride in Omaha. She never heard from him and believed him dead. "Because if he were alive he would surely come back to me," the woman said. "Our love was a great one."

This is the story told in Mrs. Hall's petition filed through Attorney Harry Hunt, wherein she is seeking to have Hall declared legally dead so that she may collect $1,000 in life insurance.

On July 26, 1921, three months after their marriage, Hall came home to her, melancholy and depressed. He had a good job, and the wife could not understand. "About 9 o'clock, said the wife, "he took up his hat and said he was going to a movie. He never came back." Mrs. Hall came to California with their son, Jack, 4 years ago. She said she had made every effort to locate Hall.

Before Jack Newton Ignatius Hall grew up and became a civil engineer, he was Mary Hall's little Jackie. One can only imagine what that was like. She had balls or, as my son, Duke, would say, "a big old nut sack." Before Dad sliced and diced the land for housing developments in Orange County during the sixties and seventies, he was just a kid with his nose pressed against a window, watching his mother play poker until midnight in one of the gambling boats off Catalina. Before he spearheaded the design of curbs and gutters that kept water flowing safely to storm drains, he was also a high diver on the USC diving team. As an adult, Jack Hall took pride in severing the earth into blocks of mathematical reason.

Sometimes I wonder if Dad decided to become a civil engineer because it gave him the illusion that he could change something as big and unpredictable as the earth. As a boy he learned he would never be able to change his mother. Mary Hall was never going to hold him tight, or praise him, or wipe away his tears. Closeness wasn't in the cards. Maybe that's why he turned his efforts to that other mother, Mother Earth. Now that I think about it, it helps me understand how Dad related, or didn't relate, to Mom and us kids.

Once in a while he would try to inject himself into Dorothy's inner circle: us. After all, he was our father. But how was it possible to fit in with his hard-to-understand children and his high-strung, sensitive wife? Every night Dad came home to his family, and every night we'd stop what we were doing as soon as he walked through the door and present a friendly if distant wall of silence. I'm sorry to say we never extended an invitation to join us. Dad seemed to accept it, just as he'd accepted it from his mother.

Three Stories

Dad told us kids exactly three stories about growing up, and no more. There was the story about how when he was little he had rickets so bad he had to wear braces. There was the story about how Grammy Hall made him play the clarinet in Colonel Parker's marching band, even though he couldn't stand the clarinet. And there was his favorite story: the story about meeting Mom at a Los Angeles Pacific College basketball game when they were nineteen, and how he knew right then and there that she was the only woman in the world for him. Dad's ending was always the same: "Six months later your Mudd and I eloped in Las Vegas." And that was it. Or, as Mary would say, the past schmast.

Three Memories

When I was nine, Dad taught me how to open a pomegranate. He took a knife, sliced around the circumference, laid his hands on either side, and popped it open. Inside was a chestful of garnets—my birthstone. I bit into the pomegranate. Fifty red gems came crashing into my mouth all at once. It was like biting into both heaven and earth.

There wasn't a family excursion that didn't lead to the ocean. It didn't matter if we were camping in Guaymas, or Ensenada, or up the coast past Santa Barbara; every evening Dad would sit down and stare into his acquiescent friend, the Pacific Ocean. Evening was Dad's designated few moments of peace. As I got older, I would join him with a glass of 7Up with ice. We would sit in silence. Then: "Your mother sure is a beauty." "Your Mudd—God, do I love her or what?" "Di-annie, do me a favor and be sure to tell your mother what a delicious meal she made." Compliments were Dad's way to whitewash his guilt about Mom's submissive role. He worried about Dorothy, just not enough to change the way he went about living with her. He never contemplated a different approach. As he stared into the ocean, he must have tossed a lifetime of apologies into its silence. Maybe he thought the tide would wash his troubles away.

I thought I was dying. I couldn't breathe. Asthma was bad enough, but this whooping-cough thing was way worse. When Dad turned me upside down, I got my breath back almost instantaneously. It was like a miracle. Mom was so worried, she kept me out of school for two months of my fourth-grade year. Every day she spread Vicks VapoRub on my chest, and she gave me 7Up with ice hourly. Sometimes she'd even let me watch TV. One night Dad and I saw a drama about a really old lady whose Seeing Eye dog was run over by a truck. I asked Dad why God let a dog die for nothing. He told me not to be scared. That seemed weird, because I'd heard Mom tell Auntie Martha that Dad passed out when he got pricked by a rose earlier that afternoon. I never thought of Dad as a fraidy-cat. After all, he'd saved my life. And it seemed mean of God to let the really old lady on

TV lose her dog when she was going to die soon enough anyway. So I asked Dad, "Why do old people have to die just because they're old?" He put me on his lap and said, "Old people have already had long lives, so they're prepared for death. Don't worry, they're fine, Di-annie." He gave me a kiss, put me down, and told me to get ready for bed. That night I heard Mom and Dad talking behind closed doors. Maybe Dad felt safe with Mom, safe enough to tell her about scary things like roses that made him faint, or the story of a beloved dog dying from a stupid accident, or just being old.

Think Positive

Dad found his version of the Bible, well, two bibles, in Norman Vincent Peale's *The Power of Positive Thinking* and Dale Carnegie's *How to Win Friends and Influence People.* I guess that's why he talked in clichés peppered with catchphrases like "think positive." As a girl, I repeated it over and over in hopes that I would learn to think and also be positive. When I asked Dad why it didn't seem to do any good, he'd always say, "Try again." But what was positive? And, even more important, what was think? I wanted to know. As usual he told me to keep asking, and as usual I followed his advice.

We moved into the beige board-and-batten tract home surrounded by acres and acres of orange groves at 905 North Wright Street, Santa Ana. It was 1957. The utopia Southern California held out to those of us who grew up in the fifties was irresistible. We believed happiness would come from owning a Buick station wagon, a speedboat, and a Doughboy swimming pool. It didn't take long before the orange groves started disappearing in favor of more developments, with names like Sun Estate Homes. Leveling the Orange out of Orange County made me sad, and I told Dad. His response was concise. "That's life, Diane, that's the way the cookie crumbles." In my own misbegotten way, I bought into his belief of living out the American dream, but the loss of the orange trees lingered.

The move to Santa Ana was my prelude to adolescence. Not only was I going to be a young woman; Dad started telling me how pretty I'd be and how some boy would love me all up, and wouldn't that be fun? I didn't want any boy loving me, not at all, not for a second. I began to formulate how much better it would be if a lot of people loved me instead of one confusing, hard-to-understand boy. This barely realized notion, among others, unwittingly helped drive me toward acting. Many of Dad's messages became justifications for seeking an audience in lieu of intimacy. Intimacy, like drinking and smoking, was something you had to watch out for. Intimacy meant only one person loved you, not thousands, not millions. It made me think of Mom on that stage at the Ambassador Hotel and Dad's unhappiness about having to share her with others.

We found our way to better conversations after I won a debate at Willard Junior High School. Thus began many nightly discourses over solutions to family problems and local politics. Dad was a Republican. He argued for lower taxes and better behavior. Mom, a determined Democrat, believed in higher taxation and more leniency with us kids. I chose to argue in her defense. What happened in the heat of our deliberations became a determining factor in my future. The more intense things became, the better I argued my point. Following my impulses did something wildly exciting; it triggered thought. Fighting for something within the safety of a formal context became my path to personal expression, but, more important, it gave me the opportunity to know Dad in a different way. He was a great debater. And fun too. It wasn't the subject or the content of our deliberations; it was the shared experience that meant so much. I couldn't care less if I lost. I didn't know it at the time, but this was a turning point in my relationship with my dad. I was learning how to navigate something new: Dad's mind.

C-Minus

In my fourteenth year, Mom handed me "My Diary" after a parent-teacher meeting in the eighth grade. It was her way of addressing my C-minus in English. I had been put in the so-called dumbbell section, with bilingual Mexican girls, bad boys, and drifty dreamy types like me. Bound together by a lack of skills, the buxom Mexican girls and I became friends. They took prepubescent, big-personality Diane under their wing. They were kind and generous and a great audience to my pratfalls. After three years in remedial English, I still didn't know a conjunction from a preposition or a proper noun from a common noun. In those days there were no alternative teaching methods to help kids like us. I had a lot of feelings, but I didn't understand what we were being taught. Were we even being taught? I don't think so. I think we were being "dumped." Mom was not a stickler for homework. She was more comfortable addressing my aspirations. For example, it was her idea to black out my teeth when I auditioned for the talent show with "All I Want for Christmas Is My Two Front Teeth." When I was a Melodette, she advised me to approach Mr. Anderson, our choirmaster, about singing duets like "Anything You Can Do I Can Do Better" before trying to convince him I could handle "When the Red Red Robin Comes Bob Bob Bobbin' Along" as a solo. Mom encouraged all of my performing-based activities, but that parent-teacher meeting must have convinced her that "My Diary" would help teach me to respect the power of words.

Dear Diary,

I wish I had a boyfriend. Boys are never going to like me because I'm flat. Well, maybe one boy might, but I'm not sure. There's Joe Gibbins, but he got caught sniffing glue today. Man. That's really getting bad. I hope I never know another boy who does that. Not ever.

I wish I could sing like Megan. She gets to take lessons with Kenny Akin. And she gets all the solos too. Of course everyone thinks she's neat. I'm going to ask Mom to let me take vocal lessons with Kenny Akin too. He puts on a lot of shows in Orange County.

Dear Diary,

Today, I went downtown with Virginia Odenath and Pat Amthor. All they did was talk to each other. Plus Pat told Virginia I like Larry Blair. I cannot stand one thing about her or her big fat mouth. And then of course Virginia couldn't wait to tell me Larry likes Genene Seeton. Well, he can just have her. Not only that, some person predicted the world will end tomorrow, and I got a D on my Algebra test.

One good thing though, Mom said yes to the lessons. So, I'll be singing with Megan at last. This is so neat.

Dear Diary,

I just don't think it's fair that Kenny Akin never lets me have a chance at a solo. I'm just a nothing around there. That's for sure. Maybe my time hasn't come yet. Oh well.

Dear Diary,

Today I found out that Megan is adopted, and her sister went insane and tried to kill herself. It was so sad. Why would anyone want to die? I wish no one ever had to die in the first place. It's too scary. I pray to God that in heaven everyone is happy and can't remember what it's like to wish they wanted to kill themselves like Megan's sister.

Dear Diary,

I finally got the nerve to ask a boy to the Girls Ask Boys dance. And he said he would go with me. Isn't that neat? He's in the popular crowd. He's scads of fun. He always calls me "stupid." Guess who it is? Ronnie McNeeley. I can't wait to tell Mahala Hoien, my new

best friend. His shirt size is 18. This is just about the
neatest thing ever. The girls are supposed to make the
boys a shirt that matches their blouse. Isn't that just so
cool?

Dear Diary,

The worst thing of all was the Girls Ask Boys
dance. I thought it would be a blast. But it wasn't. Ronnie acted like he was too good for me. He even asked
Pat Amthor to dance instead of me. And he had the
nerve to leave before the whole thing was over. I dispise
(spell) him. He should have at least danced with me
once. It's awful. Boys just don't like me. I'm not pretty
enough.

Dear Diary,

For Christmas Kenny put on a production called
Amahl and the Night Visitors. Megan was the lead.
Boy, does everybody primp over her or what? For in-
stance, Judy says, "Megan, are you cold?" Virginia says,
"Megan, here, take my coat." Meanwhile, I'm freezing.
Do you think they'd offer me their coat?

Kenny had a long talk with me today and said that
he would be using me a lot next year. And that someday
I'd be a great comedian. Har de har.

Kenny Akin

Kenny Akin was known as "Mr. Music of Orange County."
He looked like a six-foot-four version of Howdy Doody
without Buffalo Bob pulling the strings. Even though I
couldn't process the meaning of my student-teacher relationship with this larger-than-life character, I must have
instinctively known he was a means to an end. Besides
producing and directing *Kismet, Oklahoma!,* and *Babes in
Toyland,* Kenny Akin managed his own voice-and-dramatics
studio and portrayed leading tenor roles in numerous pro-
ductions from Los Angeles to San Bernardino County. Kenny's protégée, Megan, and I were both thirteen, but Megan
was poised and attractive and had an all-out killer voice. No
getting around it: Kenny thought Megan was as close to perfection as a person could be. In his eyes I was one thing
only—WRONG.

Thank God he never bought into my brand of appeal.
His rejection gave me the will to persist long enough to find
a loophole that would force him to give me a chance. As
always, my loophole was Mom. Over a cup of coffee at the
kitchen counter, I told her how Kenny gave all the big parts
to Megan. Mom didn't say anything; she just shook her
head. But I know for a fact she had a little chat with Mr.
Akin, because a few days later I saw them through a crack
in his study door. All I can say is Dorothy Deanne Keaton
Hall could be very convincing when it came to her children.

After Mother's chat, I was assigned bit parts that led to

Raggedy Ann in *Babes in Toyland*. I must have scored big, because Kenny started to take me more seriously. That's when I started to take him less seriously. It wasn't long before I told Mother I didn't want to study with Kenny anymore. I'd learned all I needed to know from him. I couldn't articulate my thoughts, but with enough experience under my belt, I'd learned how to hold my own at least long enough to find my way to an audience. The audience would decide my fate, not Mr. Kenny Akin. I always thought I'd be crushed by people who didn't buy into me. But I wasn't. There would be many Kenny Akinses who found themselves stuck with me whether they liked it or not.

Applause

There was no discussion with my parents on the night I sang "Mata Hari" in our Santa Ana High School production of the musical *Little Mary Sunshine*. Under the direction of our drama teacher, Mr. Robert Leasing, the production was worthy of Broadway—at least, that's what it was like for me. I was Nancy Twinkle, the second lead, who loves to flirt with men. Little did I know that her big song, "Mata Hari," would be a showstopper. I ran around the stage singing about the famous spy "who would spy and get her data by doing this and that-a," ending with a grand finale featuring me sliding down a rope into the orchestra pit. That was when I heard the explosion. It was applause. When Mom and Dad found me backstage, their faces were beaming. Dad had tears in his eyes. I'd never seen him so excited. More than excited—surprised. That's what it was. I could tell he was startled by his awkward daughter—the one who'd flunked algebra, smashed into his new Ford station wagon with the old Buick station wagon, and spent a half hour in the bathroom using up a whole can of Helene Curtis hairspray. For one thrilling moment I was his Seabiscuit, Audrey Hepburn, and Wonder Woman rolled into one. I was Amelia Earhart flying across the Atlantic. I was his heroine.

Later, Dad would boast about my career, but it was "Mata Hari" that became our watershed moment. There were no words. It was all—every timeless second—encapsulated in his piercing light-blue eyes. The ones Mom fell in love with. There was no going back.

PART TWO

3
MANHATTAN

The Neighborhood Playhouse

I don't remember getting on the plane that took me three thousand miles away from home when I was nineteen. I don't remember what I was wearing or what the flight was like. I don't remember kissing my family goodbye. I remember the bus ride to the city. I remember the YWCA. It was on the West Side. I remember checking in to a tiny room. I remember sitting on the stoop, watching people rush past buildings. I was in the city of my dreams. Every New Year's Eve I'd sat in front of our twenty-one-inch Philco Predicta television set and watched the ball drop in Times Square. New York was wall-to-wall mile-high buildings. It was the opposite of dinky Santa Ana or even Los Angeles. It was Times Square, the Empire State Building, the Statue of Liberty, and the Chrysler Building too. But most of all it was New Year's Eve.

It was hundreds of thousands—no, millions—of people gathered together to celebrate the ringing in of a new year. I wanted to stand with them too, right there, right in front of the Broadhurst Theatre, where hits like *Pal Joey, Auntie Mame,* and *The World of Suzie Wong* played to packed houses. New York was movies too, movies like *Breakfast at Tiffany's.* It was Audrey Hepburn with the endless cigarette holder dangling from her perfect mouth. New York was my destiny; I was going to study at the Neighborhood Playhouse School of the Theatre. I was going to be an actress. And I was ready. That's when the doorman came over and told me not to sit in front of the Y. That's all I remember: the city, the room, how ready I was, and "Don't sit on the stoop."

At the Neighborhood Playhouse, it was Sandy Meisner. He wore a camel's hair coat. He smoked and everyone said he was homosexual, even though he'd been married. I'd never heard of a married man who was gay but looked straight. He was mesmerizing and mean and the first grown man I ever thought of as sexy. I loved the ashes that were as long as the cigarette that dangled from his mouth. I loved how they fell onto his camel's hair coat. I couldn't take my eyes off him. He was the most exotic man I'd ever seen.

In Mr. Meisner's acting class, there were no accolades. Things didn't go like that. To Sandy, acting was about reproducing honest emotional reactions. He felt that the actor's job was to prepare for an "experiment that would take place onstage." His approach was designed "to eliminate all intellectuality from the actor's instrument and to make him a spontaneous responder," which could be learned by practicing the Repetition Game. It went like this. A partner—let's say Cricket Cohen—would make an observation about me. "Diane, you have brown hair." I listened and repeated the sentence she spoke. "I have brown hair." Observing some aspect of my hair, Cricket might say, "Your brown hair is also straight and thin." I would respond with something like, "Yes, my hair is straight and thin." She would embellish, adding, "Very thin." I would reply, "You're right, it is thin, very thin, but not curly like yours." The implication being, "You got a problem, asshole?" She would respond, "At least my hair is not *too* thin." Meaning something to the effect of, "Lay off, bitch. Go back to Santa Ana where you belong." And on and on, until we both ended up expressing a variety of emotions based on our reactions to each other's behavior. I took to the Repetition Game like a fish to water.

Sandy Meisner also introduced us to the world of playing with our feelings, especially the embarrassing ones. I learned to use my suppressed anger to good effect. I could cry on a dime, explode, forgive, fall in love, fall out, all in a matter of moments. My weakness? I was "too general." At the end of the second year, he cast me as Barbara Allen in *Dark of the Moon*. Rehearsals were fraught with anxiety. One day I entered stage right, singing, "A witch boy from the mountain came, a-pinin' to be human, for he had seen the fairest gal, a gal named Barbara Allen." Meisner yelled as only he could, "Why are you traipsing around like you're Doris fucking Day?"

Sandy taught us to respond to our partner's behavior. End of discussion. He forced us to hang in with the truth of the moment. No questions. He made observing and listening a prelude to expression. Point-blank. He was simple and direct. Without embellishing, he gave us the freedom to chart the complex terrain of human behavior within the safety of his guidance. It made playing with fire fun. I loved exploring the shared moment, as long as Sandy was watching. There was one cardinal rule: "Respond to your partner first, and think later." If you broke that rule, he would start laying on the one-liners. "There's no such thing as nothing." "In the theater, silence is an absence of words, but never an absence of meaning." "May I say as the world's oldest living teacher, 'Fuck polite!'" More than anything, Sandy Meisner helped me learn to appreciate the darker side of human behavior. I always had a knack for sensing it but not yet the courage to delve into such dangerous, illuminating territory.

The First Year

Dear Family,

The Rehearsal Club is on 53rd Street, right down the block from the Museum of Modern Art. I wish you could see it. It's an old brownstone. All I can think of is how lucky I am to be rooming with Pam, who is also a new student at the Neighborhood Playhouse. Thank you so much for helping me out. I feel safe, and there's a lot of other young women who live here, like Sandy Duncan, who is my age but already works professionally, I think as a dancer. All us gals share a phone down the hall. The Rockettes hog it. They have more money, I guess, or maybe they're just lonely. I don't know.

They work hard, and look hard too. Probably because of all that makeup they wear. I wouldn't want to be a Rockette for all the money in the world.

School is intense. From 9–5 every day. Wow! I'm very pleased to be working with my partner, Cricket Cohen. She's excellent to play off of. We practice all the time, and we seem to be doing well. I hope so anyway.

By now, Dorrie's either a Willard Junior High School cheerleader or not. I hope she got it. Why isn't Randy dating anyone yet? What's happening with Robin besides the fact she gave up flag twirling for homework? Wow! Oh, well, I've got to study my lines for this scene from Clifford Odets's *Waiting for Lefty*. Keep sending photographs. I miss you all.
Love, Diane

Hey, Everyone,

Can't get to sleep tonight. I feel like I've had 5 or 6 cups of black coffee. I got the money you sent. Thank God. Only one more month of the Rehearsal Club, and Pam. I don't think I should say it like that; I mean, sharing a room has been a real learning experience. I just can't wait to get home for summer. I'm really nervous about whether I'll get asked back for the second year. What if I don't?

I'm here sitting in class doing nothing because my partner, Bernie, hasn't learned his lines. What a waste of time. Bernie is so annoying. If Mr. Meisner thinks our

scene is lousy, it's going to hurt my chances for next
year. He already got rid of Laura, who happened to be
really amazing. Do you think I should ask for a new
partner? Or would that make me a creep? If I lay into
Bernie, it's not going to do any good. And anyway, he's
completely nuts.

How is everyone? What's new? Has Domino still
got too many fleas? Is Randy shaving yet? How are the
pimples on Robin's forehead? And what about Dorrie
Bell? Everything still fit as a fiddle?
Take care,
Love, Diane

The Second Year

Dear Mom,

I can't stand it. The second year is so much harder.
Mr. Meisner is really pushing us to expand into interpretation. I don't know how to create a character. I understand the repetition exercise, but being someone
else? And everyone's so much more competitive this
year. Nobody is sloughing off. It makes me nervous.
Meisner keeps telling us we have to be more specific. As
you know, that's the area I have the most trouble. We're
performing singing scenes for the 1st year soon. You'll
never guess what I'm doing. MR. SNOW from *Carou-
sel*. Again? I'm sick of Mr. Snow. In acting class we're
doing Restoration scenes, which is by far beyond me.

See you in a month. I can't wait to come home for
Christmas.
Much love,
Diane

Mr. and Mrs. Jack N. Hall:
The Neighborhood Playhouse School of the
Theatre cordially invites you to attend *Dark of the
Moon,* a program to demonstrate the work now
in progress, February 16 and 17, 1967.

Mom and Dad . . . Doesn't this crack you up? They
sent this to me instead of you. Get back here quick so
you can come see it. I hope you like my interpretation
of Barbara Allen. I sing that Joan Baez song. It's beautiful. Richard Pinter is brilliant as the Witch Boy. I hope a
lot of agents come.
Love,
Diane

And they did. The several agents who came seemed interested, but no one signed me up. At the end of my two years
at the playhouse, Sandy Meisner sent me into the world of
auditions with a nod, saying, "Someday you're going to be a
good actress."

Hair

After the Neighborhood Playhouse, I hung out with other second-year students who were panicked about the future. We didn't know where we would live, much less how to become working actors. Richard Pinter, my *Dark of the Moon* co-star, became a very close friend. Sarah Diehl and Nola Safro were around, and so was Guy Gillette, whose band, the Roadrunners, occasionally featured me singing songs like Aretha Franklin's "Respect." (Insane, and a complete disaster.)

Luckily, Hal Baldridge from the playhouse got me a job at the Woodstock Playhouse, where I appeared in *The Pajama Game* and *Oh! What a Lovely War*. It was the Summer of Love, and somehow I met my first famous man, Peter Yarrow of Peter, Paul and Mary and "If I Had a Hammer" fame. He sort of took me under his wing for a couple of days. We were hanging out at his manager Albert Grossman's place. I had no idea Peter was a political activist who organized peace festivals or that he marched with Martin Luther King. I felt awkward and uninformed with such sophisticated people and left early. He must have known I wasn't ready for the big time, because I never heard from him again. To be so close to stardom and so far away was exciting but challenging and disappointing at the same time.

When I got my Actors' Equity card, it was the end of Diane Hall. Apparently there was a Diane Hall in good standing. I decided to use Dorrie's name instead of Di, Danielle, or Dede Hall for the part of "Factory Worker" in *The*

Pajama Game. Snapping out of what must have been a self-induced stupor, I realized it was ludicrous to borrow my sister's name, so I became Cory Hall for the stellar role of "Ensemble" in *Oh! What a Lovely War.* Cory and Dorrie? That's when it dawned on me I could keep it all in the family by using Mom's maiden name. Keaton. Diane Keaton.

Dear Gang,

    I had an audition last night for a rock musical called *Hair.* I go back tomorrow for the final elimination. I've got my fingers crossed. I really hope I get it. I'm also supposed to try out for some sort of TV pilot, which doesn't pay unless it sells. We'll see.

    I'm frantically looking for an apartment, but it's so hard. The cheap ones go fast, even though they're located in the worst, most rotten areas. Today I went to the Upper West Side. No luck. I'm thinking of going to a real estate broker. I know, I'll have to pay a fee, but in the long run it's probably better. This is more of a hassle than I expected.

    Dorrie and Robin, I've started listening to Tim Buckley and Mimi and Richard Fariña. Are you into them?

Love,

Diane

Hello, all you Halls,

    We're in our 2nd week of rehearsal. Things are shaping up slowly, but I suppose that's part of it. Get ready, it's a really weird show, to put it mildly. I have three verses of a solo in a song called "Black Boys." I'm just glad I haven't been fired yet! Acting doesn't seem to be a concern to the director, Tom O'Horgan. We look like hippies; we sing like hippies; we're the turned-on youth of today. It doesn't really appeal to me! I just wish I had more to do in the show.

Anyway, I love you all.

Diane

Hi, Everyone,

Well, I'm in a hit, we opened the 29th. No Woodstock this summer. A real job, and on Broadway.

After the show tonight, Richard Avedon is photographing the whole cast for *Vogue* magazine. Now, is that astonishing or what? And big stars have come to see it, like Warren Beatty (remember my crush on him from *Splendor in the Grass*) and Julie Christie, who is the most beautiful woman I've ever seen, and Liza Minnelli, and Terence Stamp, and Carol Channing. Apparently *Hair* is the in thing to see. People stand in lines every day to get tickets.

Things are pretty much the same. I'm certainly the same. Will I ever change? I'm still the dumbest person alive. One apparently does not grow out of stupidity. Oh, also I'm on a diet. Obese is an understatement. I've gotten carried away with the FOOD LIFE.

Dad, I hope you prepared your friend for *Hair* and the nudity. Is he coming soon?

Love, Diane

4

BIG YEAR

"Father Mother"

While I was watching fellow tribe members shed their clothes onstage every night, Mom switched from letters to journals. It was 1969. She had gone from a twenty-four-year-old woman feeling the newness of two loves, to an adoring mother who reaped the so-called "rewards" of being a home-maker in the fifties, to an adult who displayed hints of defiance in the sixties.

The process of learning how to explore her own unanswered questions came from the action of moving a pen across paper. How had she found time? Not while preparing the endless tuna casseroles and cheese enchiladas that became leftovers for four lunch boxes five days a week; not at the kitchen counter, with wilting Kellogg's Corn Flakes sprinkled with wheat germ waiting to be cleared. When was she able to grab a few minutes for herself? Not after Dad was at work or we were in school; not before figuring out the best way to stretch the budget so she could buy the extras everybody always begged for. Did she have free time between the dishes and laundry, and mending our clothes, and renewing her license, and helping Dorrie with her homework? No.

I have free time, time enough to have written this memoir while working on a product line for Bed Bath & Beyond and editing a book for Rizzoli Publications on modern architecture, time to leave home and act in a Larry Kasdan low-budget indie in Park City, Utah.

Even though Dexter, Duke, and I carry on the Hall family tradition of sitting down to dinner every night, our "It takes a village" version of the evening meal is unrecognizable from those days at the kitchen counter on Wright Street. My role as "Father Mother" (coined by Duke) is nothing like Mom's. I reside at the head of the table. Dexter and Duke flank me on either side. Members of Team Keaton attend, like Sandra Shadic—renamed Sance Underpants by Duke— on some nights, "La La" Lindsay Dwelley on others. Ronen Stromberg comes by too. I love our dinners, but I don't make them. Debbie Durand does.

As "Father God" (another of Duke's terms of endearment), I begin with the high points and low points of our collective day. Duke makes a face. I pretend to ignore it and attempt to expand our sense of community spirit by injecting subjects like Heal the Bay's annual report card on the worst beaches of Southern California. Dexter says, "At least it wasn't Santa Monica again." "Right, Dex. Thank God." On the sidelines, Duke teases Dexter about her interchangeable crushes on boys with names like Max and Matthew and Tyler and Corey and Chris B. and Chris L. Dexter responds by calling Duke an "annoying pest" and ratting him out, saying Duke's school pants got thrown into the shower after swim practice by him, not by Sawyer, as he claimed. Sandra reminds her to "give your brother a break." I end it with "Duke Keaton! Sorry, but, guess what? Fun freeze." Things get better when we begin the chat about Dexter's high point, her birthday dinner. She wants fried onion rings, chicken nuggets, buttered pasta, the tuxedo cheesecake from the Cheesecake Factory, and no GREEN of any kind at all whatsoever. Everyone joins in the cleanup. Dexter wants to use my iPhone. I give it to her reluctantly and begin talking about Elizabeth Edwards's tragic ending, even quoting a sentence from the *New York Times* obituary about "the disparity between public image and private reality." No one responds. Sandra, the fastest draw in the west, has put all the plates in the dishwasher before I can begin to get the milk to the refrigerator.

Mother's time opened up when I left for New York City and Randy got a job as an usher at the Broadway Movie Theater in Santa Ana. Dorrie and Robin were wrapping up their high school years as Mother sat down and began to explore her thoughts on paper. It took the beginning of an end, on the cusp of the next decade, before Dorothy found her voice.

New Year's Eve, 1968

I'm so excited for Robin; she got a job at Bullock's as a demonstrator for cosmetic items. Dorrie is taking a ceramics class in Placentia. Jack and I have two Schwinn bikes we ride every other night to Baskin and Robbins 31 Flavors in Honer Plaza. So much fun. Randy's writing more than ever. I'm so proud of him. Jack won the best speaker award at Toastmasters. Randy goes too and loves it. Diane's coming home for a week. She got a break from rehearsals for Woody Allen's Play It Again, Sam. *Apparently she'll be going to Hollywood for some auditions. She is now a light blond, very thin young woman. The total look is extremely GOOD! Everyone remarks about our beautiful daughters.*

I started painting the kitchen. Jack's almost got the fireplace mantel finished. It makes the whole room look just the way we want it: rustic, warm, and light. I can't believe it's all working out so well. I finished my first paid photo assignment today: 20 shots of Judy Weinhart in a book for $35.00. I hate to admit I'm pretty pleased. But I am.

I took a long ride in the industrial part of Santa Ana and had the greatest time looking at old rusty tin cans, wind-blown bottles, pitted rocks, toppled shacks, and torn signs. It was as if I could SEE the silence. Today Jack said that even if I divorced him, he would come home every night. . . . I loved that because that's our story; we are infinitely tied to one another.

Thank you, somebody! Everybody. Thank you, Randy,

Robin, Dorrie, Diane, and Jack. Thank you, people, nature, animals, Goya, and Kernel, our cats. We have so much. I feel my life is very full of beauty and love. Lets see if 1969 can be even better.

January 30, 1969

Dear Mom,

I moved yesterday; what a job! I wonder what it would be like if I actually had some furniture. Thanks for the box of goodies. I love the great teapot and the photographs. They're fantastic. There's no real place to put them except on the windowsill, which compensates for the LOUSY original stove. At least my stereo works. I've been playing Nina Simone and Morgana King, my favorite.

The rehearsals are going okay. Woody Allen is cute and, of course, very funny.

I know Dad wanted me to write down all my ideas concerning the money I owe him. Certainly I'm in no position to pay it all back right now. The landlord informed me that I owe him 29 dollars, and the telephone bills will be coming soon. When the play opens I want to take singing and dancing lessons. But tell Dad not to worry because next month I'm going to start to send 50 dollars every month until I pay back the 500 dollars I owe him. In the meantime, here's my list of my expenses.

1. Rent $98.32. 2. Phone $10.00. 3. Phone service $5.00. 4. Singing lessons $40 a month, I guess. (Ugh.) 5. Dancing lessons $30, about. 6. Food $100 a month (I

guess). That's a total of $283 and 32 cents. It seems like an awful lot.

Love,

Diane

February 6, 1969

Jack and I flew all the way to New York City for the opening night of Play It Again, Sam. *Jack Benny—Ed Sullivan— Walter Kerr—George Plimpton—Angela Lansbury—and other stars attended. We met Woody Allen afterwards. Oh my goodness. He was so shy and quiet, not like I expected at all. The play was very funny. Diane looked beautiful onstage—she wore a fall, which made her hair look really thick. She's on a thing these days, always chewing a big mouthful of Dubble Bubble gum or sucking candy—or eating. I wish I knew how she stays so thin.*

Everyone was very kind to us. At Sardi's we sat at a table for 10 with champagne and cheesecake. We were told that Woody Allen's new leading lady was his new heart interest too. This gave us a real kick.

February 10, 1969

We're back home. I'm taking a class at UCI. My goal is to work HARD on writing an article and SELL IT. According to my teacher, if you want to write, write. Maybe I could work on something personal yet universal, like the way the kids are growing up so fast? I don't know.

Seeing Diane was an experience. I can't think of how to explain her effect on people. Of course, I'm speaking as I see her and am not without total bias. She is a mystery. She is independent. At times she's so basic, at others so wise it frightens me that I got so far in this world without the benefit of such knowledge. I miss her.

February 18, 1969

Dear Mom,

It seems like you were just here. How did it go by so fast? Isn't Woody hilarious? Did you really like the play? I couldn't exactly tell. Woody does a lot of let's just say unusual things onstage, things you wouldn't think a person of his stature would do. Last night, in the middle of a scene he suddenly started impersonating James Earl Jones in *The Great White Hope*. I tried not to laugh, but it was impossible.

I think I had a date with him. We went to Frankie and Johnnie's famous steakhouse. Everything was going well until I scraped my fork against the plate and made a normal, I stress normal, cutting noise. It must have driven him nuts, 'cause he yelped out loud. I couldn't figure out how to cut my steak without making the same mistake, so I stopped eating and started talking about women's status in the arts, like I know anything about women and the arts. What an idiot. The whole thing was humiliating. I doubt we'll be having dinner

together anytime soon. Today he sent me a little note. I
think you'll relate.
Love,
Diane

From Woody

Beet Head,

Humans are clean slates. There are no qualities in-
digenous to men or women. True, there is a different bi-
ology, but all defining choices in life affect both sexes &
a woman, any woman is capable of defining herself
with total FREEDOM. Therefore women are anything
they choose to be & frequently have chosen & defined
themselves greater than men. Don't be fooled by <u>THE
ARTS!</u> They're no big deal; certainly no excuse for people acting like jerks & by that I mean, so what if up till
now there were very few women artists. There may have
been women far deeper than, say, Mozart or Da Vinci
but contributing their genius in a different socially cir-
cumscribed context. Note how I switched from pen to
pencil at this moment because in Lelouch's film, A
MAN & A WOMAN, he switches from color to black
& White—So I underline my point using the same
symbolism—Very clever? OK, then, very stupid.

Woody

March 20, 1969

Diane was nominated for the Best Supporting Actress for the Tony Awards coming in April. Randy's writing teacher read two of his poems in class. One, called "Out of the Body," was submitted to the school yearbook. He'll make it.

Out of the Body

All the voices of my past are here in this grassy clearing
At the foot of the mountain.

At first I thought it was the rattle of nesting birds,
perhaps rocks falling from a cliff.
Like bells, the words took shape.

Paragraphs etched out of trees.
Stories of lives hung sadly in the air, like pages of
        failure.

I didn't want to listen
I heard my own voice on the flat face of the mountain;
        small, and weak.

I heard the sound of myself dying in the cold,
Another animal;
An animal with the gift of language
caught in the trap of distance.

June 14, 1969

Sunday night 10 p.m. The Tony Awards. Diane lost to some other gal. She was on TV, but we couldn't see her more than once, and it was fleeting.

July 7, 1969

A letter arrived from the draft board asking for verification from Randy's psychologist that he's unable to serve. It felt like a threat. Grandma Hall called. She thinks Randy was scared! Well, why not? He probably was. Who wouldn't be? "If we could learn how to prevent war, wouldn't that be enough?" he said. These are divisive times.

> July 16, 1969
> Department of the Army
> To Whom It May Concern:
> I have known Randy Hall for more than 15 years during which time I had the opportunity to observe the boy both as a neighbor and as a patient. Though he has never been mentally ill in the classical, clinical sense of the term he has demonstrated a prolonged condition of emotional instability which, in my opinion, would make him unfit for military service. Recent observation of the boy would cause me to have no change in that opinion, though he has managed to develop some cov-

ering behaviors which may have the impression of greater maturity and development than actually exists.

As a psychologist currently working with the Department of Defense in an overseas setting I believe that this boy would not fit into the military service and would actually be a liability rather than an asset to the military community.

William L. Bastendorf, PhD
Associate Director Pupil Personnel Services

More Positive Thinking

Just in case we might have been looking for a little quick advice, Dad had several copies of Dale Carnegie's *How to Win Friends and Influence People* prominently placed throughout our house on Wright Street. Part of its appeal came from clever chapter headings, categorized in sections with quick-fix nuggets. "Twelve Ways to Win People to Your Way of Thinking: 1. Avoid arguments. 2. Never tell someone they are wrong. 3. Start with a question the other person will answer yes to. 4. Let the other person feel the idea is his."

Dad's letters were an homage to Carnegie's influence. "Dear Diane, Rule 1. January 5 is one of those days that make men older. A daughter 20 years old is not really an asset to a young man like myself! Truth in government is a must, but truth in age is stupid. Starting now, you are 17 and I am 35. Love, Jack N. Hall, your father."

Next to Dale Carnegie's book was Norman Vincent

Peale's *The Power of Positive Thinking*. Published in 1952, it stayed on the *New York Times* bestseller list for 186 weeks, selling more than five million copies. The country was in love with Peale's cozy quotes. "When life hands you lemons, make lemonade." "The tests of life are not meant to break you, but to make you." "A positive mental attitude means you can overcome any kind of trouble or difficulty." Dad ate it up. He didn't give a damn about critics who claimed Peale was a fraud.

At age forty, Jack Hall quit his job as Santa Ana City Hall's civil engineer to become the president of Hall & Foreman, Incorporated. He gave credit where credit was due, claiming every bit of his business acumen had been enhanced 100 percent by applying Carnegie's and Peale's tried-and-true techniques. Mom must have been sick and tired of hearing Dad list the twelve steps he learned to be an effective leader. But guess what? Within a few years he was a self-made success.

By 1969, Dad's business was booming. Mom let her hair grow long and wore bell-bottoms. They began to drink socially. She became more liberal. He became more conservative. Even though they were attractive and, by Southern California standards, almost wealthy, it didn't make them happier.

The problems began when Dad started inserting his self-help solutions into the family dynamic, especially regarding Randy, who didn't have a firm handshake or "plan ahead" and wasn't always "positive." Toastmasters was still a form of torture for Randy, even though he told Mom he loved it.

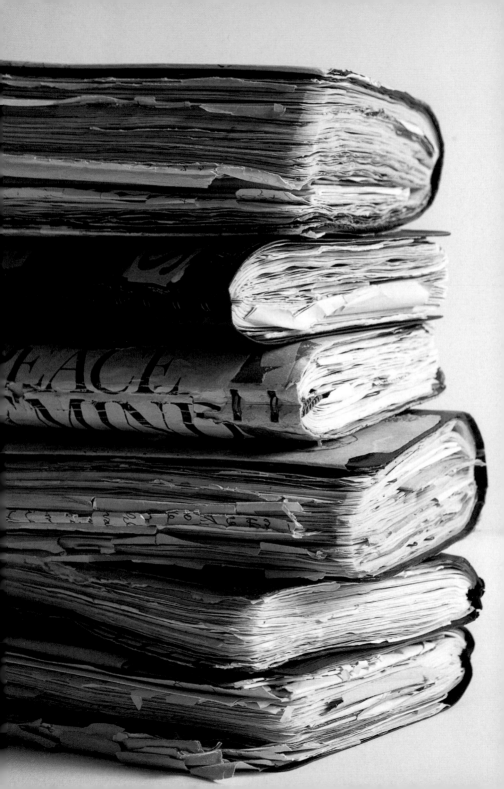

diane
keaton

Bri
Comp
PETERBROUGH
(AP) — An

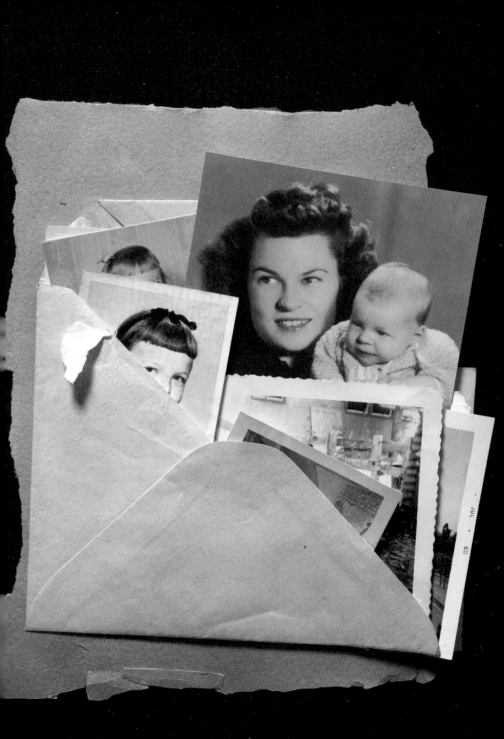

May 29. One of the days that comes as a reward
in life! It was a Thursday.
If I take it in order it will go like this:
Got up - nothing here - dreary morning - hard to
get going - glum - dumb - blah - fed-fp for-fum
Early morning duty on the playground and this
brings about a certain amount of wake-up power -
just being out in the yard at 8:10 with all those
kids. They gather round with all sorts of tales
to relate. A book could be written about these.
Then class at 8:30. Good day of doing things
together. (My biggest treat in the day is reading
their work at the end of the morning.) The
creative minds of these kids is unknown to most
everyone. It's the greatest thing in the world,
to me.
Afternoon was enacting the Three Pigs by the kids.
They are getting so good at this.
Then home - Randy came out and said he had surprises
One in the house and one in the garage. One of
the big things of greatness in my mental life is
surprises. A personal note was written to Randy
from quartet Mag. about his work. Beautiful!
Then in the kexx garage was a Honda 90 for MOM.
It's one of those easy ones anyone can ride. He
too, I can ride it and it is fun. Dorrie loves it
and w are all going riding tomorrow. Then after
that beautiful day Jan and I went out for dinner,
looking at clothes and home feeling like great
people. (We ARE!) May 29 - you were great, too.

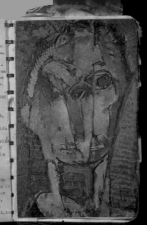

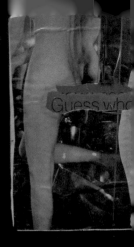

Guess who

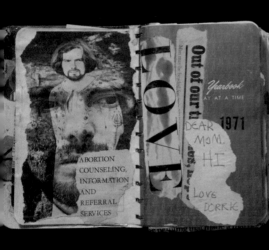

LOVE

ABORTION
COUNSELING,
INFORMATION
AND
REFERRAL
SERVICES

Out of our ti

Yearbook
DAY AT A TIME

1971

DEAR
MOM.
HI

LOVE
DORRIE

Tuesday, July 17, 1973
198th Day—167 days to follow

I'm remembering the higher
back up can like - the old
red street car where we waited in
safety zones for the limousine
to come to pick us up for off
or token or passes -

I'm remembering 1968 when I had
my first operation. I'll be thinking
of you tonight for her her
cramps - We went to N.Y. to see
Liszt in "Hair" - all of us had
job - I limped about with
sore - feet - Rickenbach
took us around - Randy - all
of us - So long ago - my mind
picks up these demon-dreams
that eat good to my mind

Ordered glasses from Boutique - N.G.
Wednesday, July 18, 1973
199th Day—166 days to follow

So
many
things
have
changed
so
quickly
I
forgot
how
fast
time
moved

AND
that
was
for
ME.

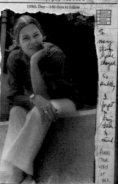

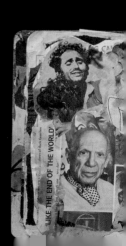

"LIKE THE END OF THE WORLD"

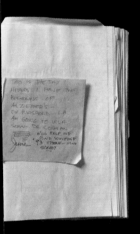

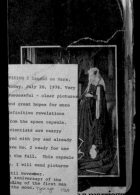

On sticky note (img near center-left):
THIS IS THE DAY I
HOPED I'D HAVE THE
BEGINNINGS OFF
ALZIEMER'S —
DR RESEARCH — LA
AM GOING TO UCLA
SOON DR CONRAD
WILL HELP ME
FIND SOMEONE
June '93 THERE — SCARY
SCARY

I am strongly influenced by
Don Juan:
"Sit quietly and let the
twilight fill you. Do whatever
you want now, but when I
tell you, look straight at those
shiny clouds and ask the
twilight to give you power
and calmness."
advice to Carlos Castaneda

wrote to "Born at Home" about
sense exchange — Had some story,
not like today — feelings of growth
in awareness that I'm aware that
I am first to recognize small steps
I work my way along — and when
I am showed my way I'm ready +
glad — change and happening all
the time — I see what Betty — in me,
in others, in habits in happening
in thoughts — all ways — I feel
my life — I really do I try want I
I have no problems or troubles for
anyone else — yet keep my self-image
felt —

I took my bath and my two cats were
stretched out on the floor beside me. It's
like they know when I relax I feel happy —
I don't want me to touch them no more —
I love the look of those two — field rather
curiously arranged + trackie so very different
so odd what it's fun looking at these fellows

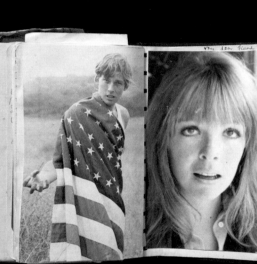

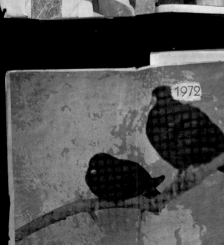

1972

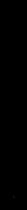

VIKING I landed on Mars,
today, July 20, 1976. Very
successful — clear pictures
and great hopes for more
definitive revelations
from the space capsule.
Scientists are teary
eyed with joy and already
have No. 2 ready for use
in the fall. This capsule
I will send pictures
until November.
anniversary of the
landing of the first man
on the moon. Tyn age 1969
a marriage

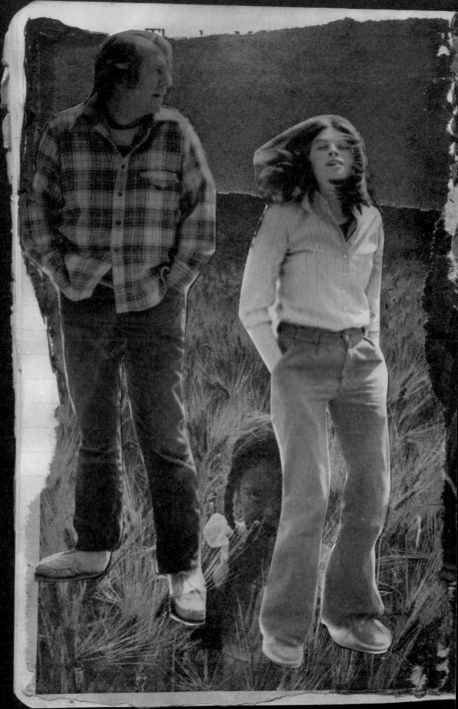

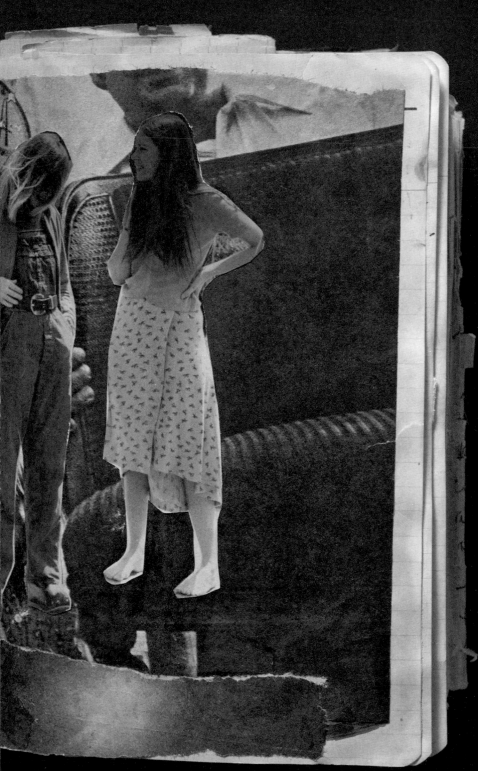

PACE

There is no record of how Dad discovered PACE, an acronym for Personal and Company Effectiveness. PACE was described as a method to help people better understand what it would take to make more productive use of their talents while further enhancing their personal and professional success. But he did. Everyone in my family went to San Diego for the two-week summits, filled with seminars guided by specialized counselors in the field; everyone except me.

Daniel Whiteside was the director of youth activities. Neither Randy, Robin, nor Dorrie has any memory of him. Years later I found his qualifications on a website, which stated that he has a master's degree in language arts from the University of California at San Francisco and the equivalent of a doctorate from the Interstate College of Personology.

Personology was developed in the 1930s by Edward Vincent Jones, a Los Angeles circuit court judge who took notes on the behavioral patterns of people who appeared in his courtroom. Judge Jones, a close friend of Whiteside's parents, eventually "proved" that he could predict people's behavior by observing their facial features. Examples of Personology correlations are: (1) Thick, unruly hair: less sensitive. (2) Thin hair: extremely sensitive. (3) Broad-jawed: authoritative in speech and action. (4) Square, angled chin: can be combative. (5) Heart-shaped jaw or chin: tends to be passive.

Randy's jaw is wide. According to the principles of Personology, that meant he was confident, assured, and domineering. Robin must have been passive and compliant because of her narrow chin. Dorrie's hair is thick and coarse. Was she really less sensitive, even though her ability to understand and share feelings for others was unusually intuitive? Did Whiteside even notice the Hall family adolescents' facial features? Or had he put aside the research required for the equivalent of a doctorate from the College of Personology? Maybe he was in the process of creating his own "Three in One Concepts."

As for James W. Newman, the founder of PACE, Dad couldn't have cared less if he was a certified psychiatrist or psychologist. He bought the package hook, line, and sinker. Dad's decision to implement the principles of PACE as a replacement for help from a genuine psychiatrist backfired, like all of his attempts to guide Randy into the responsibilities of his role as Junior Jack.

As Emmet's nephew and Mary Alice's son, Dad was attracted to impostors, swindlers, and frauds. It was part of his DNA. He didn't question Dale Carnegie and Norman Vincent Peale. The thought that they might take advantage of the average Joe's need to believe in simple solutions to complex problems never entered his mind. Ironically, Dad became successful despite being gullible. He actually had a craft and a degree from USC. Little did he know it was his hard work combined with an ingenuous manner of being honest to the point of naïve that made Hall & Foreman one of the most successful engineering firms in Orange County. His straightforward manner and lack of artifice worked wonders on everyone except his family.

August 15, 1969

Jack sent Randy to PACE for a retreat in La Jolla. Robin is going next week; Dorrie too. I just hope Jack is right and it works. He feels everyone in the family will profit from the benefits of PACE. We can't work Diane in because she's busy with her own life, but maybe later in the year.

August 22, 1969

"Hey, everybody, this is my mom and her name is Dorothy." Randy made me feel like a queen when we picked him up after a week at PACE. He said it was a sort of "mountaintop-unreal-experience that makes it hard to drop back down to the flatlands." That's where the test comes. Can "I" make it work with others who don't have PACE in their lives? "I" can if "I" try.

September 1, 1969

Robin came home from PACE. She loved it; Dorrie too. But it's a constant strain to keep PACE in practice. So many things distract us. I hope it will work and we will be better people because of our strengths. The kids are seriously hanging on to the PACE concepts. They continue to read the books and practice deep relaxation. Jack feels they've learned so much. He has a lot of confidence.

Five Against One

My siblings survived PACE. Life went on. I stayed in New York. For Dad, it was the same. Number 1: Encourage everyone by making our faults seem easy to correct. Number 2: Try to make us happy about doing what he suggested. Number 3: Ask questions instead of directly giving us orders. And number 4: Talk about his own mistakes before indirectly calling attention to ours. He gradually gave up trying. After all, it was five against one.

September 5, 1969

Diane was on Merv Griffin *tonight. She was Diane. Her walk, her laugh, her jumble of words. When she sat between Bob Hope and Merv, they teased her about dating. Bob Hope said, "All right, Diane, who is he?" She couldn't get her words out. She was nervous and giggly, but with Bob Hope next to her everything she said was unaccountably funny. He actually made a comedienne out of Diane. I can't exactly explain. Both Merv and Bob played off her all evening. I took pictures. Dad taped the whole thing.*

September 18, 1969

I worked up enough nerve to call Bowers Museum to have the director look at my photos—whew! That took courage.

I am trying to pull together enough good photographs to show him. I'm crossing my fingers.

Form Letter to Potential Magazine Editors

Mr. John C. Smith
Art Editor
XXX Magazine
(Address)
Dear Mr. Smith:
I can bring exceptional photography with strong natural character qualities to your magazine. The enclosed resume highlights a glimpse of my professional achievements in both photography and art, as well as my academic background.

The enclosed two photographs necessarily represent only a small segment of my scope of work. While I am flexible on subject matter, my emphasis on the natural persists in all my work.

I would like to accept a freelance assignment for XXXX magazine and can promise photographic excellence, not only as a photographer but also as an artist. If you are interested in seeing more of my work, please contact me. I will be happy to submit additional material on request and discuss a possible assignment for XXXX magazine.

I am looking forward to hearing from you.
Sincerely yours,
Dorothy Hall

With the letter, she included a publicity shot of the actress Diane Keaton.

November 6, 1969

I won first prize at the Orange County Fair last night for the giant collage I made with photographs of Robin and Dorrie. It was one of those thrilling experiences that give me hope. Today my new business cards arrived. I'm ready to go.

I got a letter from Diane about her appearance on Merv Griffin *last week. She needs more confidence. "By the way, I saw my spot on Merv Griffin. It was horrible. I wonder why I do these things. It's so painful to watch myself trying too hard. I didn't get* Butterflies Are Free *either. Too tall and too 'kooky'—a nice way of saying strange."*

Diane Minus-the-Hall Keaton

DIANE KEATON, Mom's massive extravaganza documenting my career from 1969 through 1984, is about as hard to grasp as Dad's belief in the healing powers of PACE. The cover, wrapped in shiny silver paper with giant black letters, spelled out my new minus-Hall name. The size alone (twenty by thirty inches) presents the kind of deliberation *DIANE KEATON* doesn't merit.

Kicking it off are two ticket stubs from *Play It Again, Sam,* glued next to a funny-looking caricature of Woody, next to a yellow Sardi's napkin, below several photographs of me with fellow cast members smiling in anticipation of good reviews. Then comes the four-page spread in *Harper's Bazaar* that makes it crystal clear I was not the model I aspired to be. Sure, it was really "cool" to have Bill King (famous for all those jumping shots of supermodels like Lauren Hutton) take the pictures, but I look strange in midair, with my huge smile revealing the gold caps my Santa Ana dentist reassured me would last a lifetime. Headlines like DIANE'S STAR ON THE RISE or ACTRESS DIANE KEATON CAN'T BE PIGEON-HOLED, with a handwritten note from Mom saying, "Barbara sent this from Cedar Rapids," seem sort of forced. First of all, who was Barbara from Cedar Rapids? And second, who cares? The awful review of my performance at the Ice House back in 1975 is a pathetic reminder of my stint as a nightclub singer. "She may be an adequate actress, but Diane Keaton is not a singer. Her musical selections are unvaried. Miss Keaton doesn't communicate with her audience. She uses oddly restricted facial expressions and poorly planned body gestures."

The headline from *Orange County People* stated, JACK HALL WAS RIGHT. HIS DAUGHTER DID GROW UP TO BE A MOVIE STAR.

Jack Hall's friends used to laugh when he said his little girl Diane would grow up to be a movie star. No one's laughing now. Not at all shy when it comes to praising their talented daughter, Jack and his wife Muriel will proudly tell anyone, "That's our daughter." Although they won't take any credit for Diane's talent ("She did it on her own"), it's entirely possible she inherited some of the moxie it takes to be a star from Muriel, who went back to college at 40 after raising four children and earned her degree with honors. Muriel has photographed a book jacket and an album cover for Woody Allen.

Muriel? Please. It's almost as if Mother closed her discerning eyes and went for *bulk;* even the loss of her first name didn't stop her from including the article. Why? To be reminded she had no identity other than as Jack Hall's wife and Diane Keaton's mother?

DIANE KEATON ends abruptly, with a two-page ad from the *Los Angeles Times* featuring photographs of Barbra Streisand, Farrah Fawcett, Liza Minnelli, Paul Newman, Burt Reynolds, John Travolta, and me smiling underneath the headline A CHANNEL 2 SPECIAL REPORT . . . STARDOM: DREAM OR NIGHTMARE? It was the perfect place for Mom to call it quits. Her daughter, the little girl who sang to the moon as she stood on the driveway of her parents' Quonset hut right off Monterey Road in Highland Park, had become a movie star.

Stardom never became a nightmare, but it wasn't what I thought it would be. How can you think a dream? Not even Dale Carnegie could do that. As I closed *DIANE KEATON,* a *Time* magazine with "A Comic Genius: Woody Allen Comes of Age" on the cover fell out, along with a newspaper article featuring a picture of her holding on to Dad's arm. The caption read, "Parents of actress Diane Keaton are not averse to discussing her." The article went on to say, "Mrs.

Hall, a stately, well-dressed woman who lets her husband do the talking when it comes to business, is more than glad to talk about her daughter, Diane. 'It isn't just Diane who is in the limelight, Jack and I are sharing in the glow too. It's been the most exciting time of my life. Everywhere we go with Diane we're mobbed.'" Mobbed? I've never been mobbed. Ever. Did Mother know what she was saying? Did she even say it?

Was it worth it? Did spending so many hours cutting and pasting the story of budding actress Diane Keaton—not Hall—ever feel like a waste of time? Why was Mother so engrossed with the process of validating my life? It's hard to know what to make of the parade of boring articles, interchangeable photographs, and pre-language quotes from me, like "Gee, I'm just so honored to even meet Betty Ford" and "Oh, yeah, sure . . . I loved the Martha Graham dance recital. Woody and I are both taking lessons with her company. It's so much fun." Didn't Mom feel embarrassed for me? Did she think cutting pictures into smaller squares and rectangles would be a different kind of healing? Was it numbing and nice? Was it a reassuring if abstract way to reflect on the joys of the past?

Our story, Mother's and mine, will always and forever lie hidden in a past that can't be untangled by looking through a parade of clippings recording the journey of a young woman who became Annie Hall.

December 31, 1969

I always say my life is this family, and that's the truth. Today was no exception. Dorrie pushed all of us to get up and take a bike ride to Baskin and Robbins, just like last year. It was so much fun. It's true when they say it's the little things that matter.

I have assessed my happiness ratio and this is the result. I am totally content whenever the ones I love are happy about something little, big, insignificant, whatever. I just don't think anyone could possibly have the same wonderful, intense, compelling feelings that I have for this family of mine.

Jack asked me if it was a good day—the last one of the year—and I have to say it was. We tried to get tickets to see True Grit *but couldn't, so Jack, Randy, Robin, Dorrie, and I went out to eat at Marsé Restaurant and then came home to watch Dick Clark ring the New Year in. "1969 was a BIG year, huh, Dad?" "Sure, Dorrie, sure." I hope the same will be said of 1970.*

5
THE LIST

Jane Fonda. Ally Sheedy. Joan Rivers. Paula Abdul. Lindsay Lohan. Sally Field. Princess Diana. Anne Sexton. Karen Carpenter. Anna Freud. Mariel Hemingway. Audrey Hepburn. Portia de Rossi. Meredith Vieira. Victoria Beckham. Kelly Clarkson. Felicity Huffman. Mary Kate Olsen. Catherine Oxenberg. Sharon Osbourne.

Sally Field and I are the same age. We're both actresses. We live and work in Los Angeles. That's where the similarities end, or so I thought. I've met Joan Rivers, Lindsay Lohan, Felicity Huffman, and even Audrey Hepburn. It didn't seem like we had much in common. I remember when Meredith Vieira interviewed me for *The View*. She was the kind of assured professional I admired. It's hard to believe we suffered from a mutual obsession. How is it possible I share a mutual past with Mary Kate Olsen, a person forty years younger and $100 million richer? Jane Fonda? *The* Jane Fonda? Come on. When I was introduced to Victoria Beckham at a party Katie Holmes gave in her honor, I couldn't begin to imagine who she was or the world she moved in. And yet each and every woman whose name is listed above shared the same secret. The difference? I chose to keep it to myself until now.

More

Looking inside the brown paper bag only to find a green apple, six pennies, four cherry suckers, and one Tootsie Roll Pop was way too disappointing. Why no Snickers or 3 Musketeers? With next to nothing to show for ringing neighborhood doorbells, shouting "Trick or treat!" in a gypsy costume, I worked the Randy front and conned him out of his candy by promising he could sleep in the top bunk for a week.

The next night I snuck into the kitchen while Mom and Dad were watching Milton Berle on TV. Just as I was about to snatch a handful of Hydrox cookies, I heard Dad's voice. "Diane?" Many tears later, I tiptoed to the hideout where I'd stuffed Randy's Halloween candy and ate the remains. No one found out.

You have to understand, Mom rarely bought brand names like Hydrox. Her budget did not include Hostess Twinkies, 7Up, Frosted Flakes, or, my favorite, Challenge Butter. Dinner, for example, was a generic affair. We ate a lot of meat loaf, spaghetti, hamburger patties with catsup, and casseroles—way too many casseroles. For dessert it was usually three oatmeal cookies apiece. Dad helped himself to as many as he wanted. Night after night I watched with envy as he ate his fill. Extra treats came at the beginning of the week. For instance, on Monday Mom gave me a whole piece of Wrigley's Doublemint gum. On Wednesday the tight allocation of resources forced her to hand out half a piece. By Saturday it was a measly quarter. I continued to twist Randy's arm, but the rewards were hardly worth it. My first real success came at Willard Junior High School, where I used my personality to convince several friends in dumbbell English to fund my need for Refresho ice cream bars and Fifty50s.

Magazines, one of my ancillary fixations, fit neatly into the mix, starting with *McCall's,* a fifties version of *Martha Stewart Living.* I had no interest in the fun activities on the back page for little girls. No, what I liked were the color pictures of smiling women selling Campbell's soup and Pond's face cream. They were pretty, and best of all they never changed. That was neat. *Life* magazine was neat too, because it told stories with photographs, but what really knocked my socks off was the first time I saw Miss Audrey Hepburn on the cover. She wasn't pretty. She was beautiful. In fact, she was perfect. I began to notice disturbing things about my eleven-year-old body. It was too big in the bathtub. I didn't like that. And people in real life weren't always attractive, even Mom. That was concerning. But, worst of all, I began to understand the troubling concept of comparison. When I compared myself to Audrey Hepburn, something was off. My features were not symmetrical. I wasn't pretty. At best, I was an affable-looking thing. Yuck. As I got older, it became painfully clear my appearance would always be a work in progress. I began to ponder solutions in the rearview mirror of our station wagon. The right side of my face was better than the left. Okay, not bad. If I kept my mouth slightly parted, I looked vulnerable. Vulnerable was good. By applying these new methods I was beautiful—well, not beautiful, pretty. Not really pretty, but attractive, definitely attractive. Along the way, I discovered fashion magazines like *Mademoiselle* and *Vogue*. They taught me to focus on my body as well as my face. I began to dress in a sixties version of hip. I wore miniskirts with white boots, and glittery box-shaped dresses, and even swinging ready-steady-go pantsuits. I painted my eyes with black liquid eyeliner, like Elizabeth Taylor in *Cleopatra*. I glued on false eyelashes and kept ratting my hair as if it would compensate for my failing face. I don't know why I thought I could pull off perfection—obviously it was absurd—but I kept trying.

All my half-baked forays into the world of beauty never held a candle to the lure of food. I was a closet glutton, waiting for a future where I would get what I wanted and MORE. That future became the present when I was cast in *Hair* just after I'd graduated from the Neighborhood Playhouse. You can imagine how wildly out of the ordinary it was to find myself gossiping with Melba Moore about whether it was true that Janice gave birth to her baby on LSD in Gerry Ragni and Jim Rado's dressing room after the show one night. *Hair* offered too many options. The entire cast was given a free trip to Fire Island, with lots of peyote. If you took your clothes off during a performance, you received a fifty-dollar nightly bonus. When *Hair* tribe member Lamont Washington died in a fire after he fell asleep with a lit cigarette while smoking in bed, the message of peace and love seemed beside the point. There was too much infighting and confusion thrust upon wildly talented yet inexperienced young people who didn't have the advantage of counseling, me included.

Instead of making friends, I retreated to Tad's Steak-house and indulged in the $1.29 steak dinner. The thing about Tad's was, I could eat all I wanted. While my cast mates were smoking grass, I was eating Carvel soft vanilla cones in between matinees and the evening show. My big break came when Lynn Kellogg, the lead, left to do an episode of *Mission: Impossible*. I filled in. After the first week, Michael Butler, the producer, called to tell me I could have the part if I lost weight. At five feet seven and weighing in at 140 pounds and gaining, I hightailed it to Dr. Paul, who, for fifty dollars a shot, would inject me with vitamins—speedy vitamins. I stuck with it long enough to lose ten pounds and land the starring role of Sheila, of "Good Morning Starshine" fame. With such good news, I rented a studio walk-up on West 82nd Street and got my first phone.

The Toilet Down the Hall

Diane's room is hard to describe. It's long and narrow. The tiny kitchen is curtained off with burlap. Inside is a blue chipped bathtub and washbasin, a stove to cook on, and a closet for clothes. The walls are collaged. A very small re-frigerator stands alone in the corner, working very hard be-

cause it needs defrosting so badly. Worst of all, she shares a toilet down the hall with three other tenants. Oh, dear. This is worrisome; so much for abandonment and discomfort.

When Mom and the kids' visit was over, it was goodbye, Dr. Paul; I saved an extra 150 dollars a week and said hello to ten pounds. What if Michael Butler came to the show? What if he saw I'd gained the weight back? What if I got fired? One night after several charbroiled steaks at Tad's, I overheard tribe member Shelley Plimpton talking about someone she knew who deliberately regurgitated in order to stay thin. How disgusting. How awful. How interesting. I have no memory of the first time I tried to throw up. I do remember taking a day here, a day there, to explore the effects. In no time at all I was committed to three unordinary meals a day. Breakfast took an hour; lunch two; dinner three, which added up to a time-consuming six hours a day spent processing food.

It was Sunday brunch at Grossingers seven days a week. It was breakfast with a dozen buttered corn muffins dipped in Chock Full o'Nuts coffee, plus three orders of fried eggs over hard with bacon, and a side of pancakes topped off with four glasses of chocolate milk. It was lunch to go, including three buttered steaks with salty charbroiled fat on the side, two and a half baked potatoes with sour cream and chives, a black-and-white malted with hot apple pie plus two chocolate sundaes with extra nuts from Schrafft's. Dinner began with a bucket of Kentucky Fried Chicken, several orders of french fries with blue cheese and catsup, and a couple of TV dinners. For dessert it was chocolate-covered almonds with a quart-size bottle of 7Up, a pound of See's Candies peanut brittle sent from home, M&Ms washed down with mango juice on ice, one Sara Lee pound cake, and three Marie Callender's frozen banana-cream pies. I learned to throw up so fast it had no effect. At first there was no problem with vomiting or its aftermath. I didn't need help stimulating the gag reflex. I had it under control. No fuss, no muss.

It was always the same: After the first too-good-to-be-true bites turned into the third and fourth, adjustments had to be made to re-create the original taste. When that didn't work, the menu reverted to reliable standbys like toasted white bread with butter and strawberry jam. When that took a dive, there was another switch, and another and another. The more I ate, the more disenchanted I was with the results. It didn't matter, because the impact of the first few bites triumphed over all setbacks.

My new life was labor intensive. Think of hauling all that food in all those brown paper bags up a flight of stairs and into the darkness of my room on West 82nd Street. Think of the tiny un-defrosted freezer/refrigerator and the yellowing cabinets slid open to an ever-changing array of canned goods and baked items. Think of me throwing my body into convulsions three times a day with a box of baking soda standing on the floor next to the toilet. It was as numbing as it was compulsive.

After six months of knocking off twenty thousand calories a day, I became hypoglycemic. I had heartburn, indigestion, irregular periods, and low blood pressure. I was dogged by sore throats. All of which created unwanted activity— namely, calls to doctors and trips to the pharmacy for over-the-counter Ex-Lax. Dr. Stanley Darrow, my dentist, found twenty-six cavities in one visit. Soon my front teeth had to be capped. More work. More pain. But worse were the psychological effects. I became increasingly isolated. I didn't think about friendships. I didn't acknowledge the shame. I was busy ignoring reality. I had work to do.

Woody Allen and I met in the fall of 1968 at the Broadhurst Theatre while I was auditioning for *Play It Again, Sam.* We read together. He was funny but not intimidating. I got the part, or, as Woody teased me and I used to say, "I created the role of Linda Christie." *Play It Again, Sam* was a showcase for Woody's talents. My husband, Dick Christie, played by Tony Roberts, and I took Allan Felix, played by Woody, under our wing. After he was dumped by his wife, we encouraged him to date. Unbeknownst to us, he was also getting help from Humphrey Bogart, who appeared to him during failed dating attempts with gorgeous women. Allan and Linda, both insecure, fell for each other.

During rehearsal, I fell for Allan as scripted but for Woody as well. How could I not? I was in love with him before I knew him. He was Woody Allen. Our entire family used to gather around the TV set and watch him on Johnny Carson. He was so hip, with his thick glasses and cool suits. But it was his manner that got me, his way of gesturing, his hands, his coughing and looking down in a self-deprecating way while he told jokes like "I couldn't get a date for New Year's Eve so I went home and I jumped naked into a vat of Roosevelt dimes." Or "I'd rather be with a beautiful woman than anything else except my stamp collection." Things like that. He was even better-looking in real life. He had a great body, and he was physically very graceful.

As in the play, we became friends. I was a good audience. I laughed in between the jokes. I think he liked that, even though he would always remind me I wouldn't know a joke if it hit me in the face. But I knew behavior, and his behavior was way more interesting to me than jokes could ever be. Woody got used to me. He couldn't help himself; he loved neurotic girls.

While I continued to try to convince him that I was more than a goofy sidekick, many of our conversations—even those centered on my favorite subject, me—were distracting. I was all too often pulled away by a commitment that overshadowed my crush on Woody Allen. For instance, let's say he wanted to see a three o'clock screening of *The Sorrow and the Pity* at 59th and Third. How could it work? There was no time to cash my paycheck and get to Woolworth's on 86th before it closed at seven P.M. I was running out of Kraft caramels, Boston baked beans, and bubble-gum cigars in assorted flavors. Besides, the 59th Street theater was too far away for us to have a chance to stop at Gristedes. It's pathetic that the demands of bulimia outshone the power of my desire for Woody, but they did.

On the surface, all was going well. Woody slowly began to see me as something more than a gal pal. Our relationship wasn't off and on, but it wasn't exactly committed either. Even then Woody was the most disciplined, hardworking, dedicated, organized, and—ironically—resilient person I'd ever met. On a daily basis, he practiced his clarinet, appeared in the play, read all the works of Tolstoy, and wrote new jokes for appearances in Vegas at Caesars or in Reno, where Frank Sinatra Jr. opened for Sir Woody of Allen at the medieval-themed Cal Neva Hotel. He was always busy, so nothing much was required of me. I moved a few things into his new penthouse apartment, but I kept my studio on 82nd. When it got broken into, the police advised me to put bars on the windows. I didn't listen. What did I care? The apartment was there for one thing only, to implement my routine.

Experts

A century ago, women struggled with mental problems like hysteria and anxiety, not bingeing. Today, mental-health experts believe bulimia is related to social class, income, education, the occupation of parents, and an introverted personality, which causes high rates of phobias, alcoholism, anxiety disorders, and panic attacks. Bulimic women differ from depressed women because they're more likely to be overweight and to have overweight parents. Apparently, parents with high expectations create an atmosphere that fosters eating disorders. Lack of parental affection is one of the main reasons bulimics soothe themselves with food.

Spare me. I can't stand the ease with which experts blame parents, especially mothers, for their teenage daughters', slash soon to be young adults', slash middle-aged women's, slash angry old ladies' food addictions. Come on. I'm sorry, but my mother was nothing if not affectionate. And, by the way, *dazed* is the word I would use to describe the effects of indulging in an eating disorder. The facts are the facts, but the reason one becomes bulimic is more complex than overweight mothers, which Dorothy was not.

Mom made every effort, particularly in the early days, to present a cheery worldview. She gave me everything I wanted—at least, as much as she could—but years of keeping things bottled up had their effect. Before I left home, the undertones in her silence were obvious. I must have been fourteen the first time I heard Mom and Dad fighting behind the closed door to their bedroom. I remember rushing to Randy's room, where I caught him stuffing *Playboy* pictures of bare-breasted women under his bed. Panicked, I asked him if he heard Mom and Dad yelling about getting a divorce. Did he? Did he? His response was to run away, leaving me with their not-so-muffled screams. Did this incident make me more susceptible to fulfilling a future of MORE, so much MORE? I don't know. Even if, early on, Mother had had the privilege of participating in the revelations of the analyst's couch, would my insatiable hunger have taken a backseat to a less pathological method of satisfying my needs? It's hard to say.

October 31, 2009, would have been her eighty-eighth birthday. Last Halloween she'd been dead for six weeks. This year it's been four hundred and nine days and nights without my mother. I thought time was supposed to heal all wounds. As I wait for Dexter to come out of swim practice, in my Tahoe Hybrid parked at the top of Santa Monica City College, overlooking the local graveyard, I can still see Daphne Merkin's plaintive face in the Polo Lounge this morning, whispering, "Diane, don't you think they'll come back to us? Don't you think they're coming back, our mothers?"

Daphne . . . I wish. I wish they would. All of them. All the mothers.

Packing It In

Woody didn't have a clue what I was up to in the privacy of his bathrooms. He did marvel at my remarkable appetite, saying I could really "pack it in." Ever vigilant and always on the lookout, I made sure he never caught me. This is not to say that Woody was oblivious to my problems. He knew how insecure I was. It must have been annoying as hell to be the brunt of my constant need for support and encouragement. After *Play it Again, Sam* closed, I couldn't get a job. It seemed like every audition was lost to either Blythe Danner or Jill Clayburgh, who weren't "too nutty." A year came and went without work. When I landed a commercial for Hour After Hour deodorant, where I wore a tracksuit and bit my husband's ear, saying, "Hour After Hour . . . it won't wear out before the day is over," I hit bottom. The bingeing was off the charts. What would Woody think if he knew my secret? Why couldn't I get a job? I kept fixating over something Lee Ann Fahey, another aspiring actress, said about "making it" before you're twenty-five. I was twenty-five. What was I going to do? It wasn't enough to be Woody's washed-out Ali MacGraw girlfriend. What was going to happen? Should I quit? Woody suggested I see an analyst named Felicia Lydia Landau.

Monday through Friday I walked up Fifth Avenue to 94th and Madison; got on the elevator of the nondescript red brick building; pressed the button to the sixth floor; made my exit, walked down the narrow hallway, and pushed the buzzer outside Dr. Landau's office. When she opened the door, I would say hello and hit the couch. Once on my back, with the ceiling as my horizon, I was ready to map out the history of my neurosis. We couldn't have been a more unlikely pair—me, the firstborn daughter of a sunny-looking family from Southern California; she, a Jew from Poland who escaped on the eve of Hitler's invasion.

After another year of throwing up, intermittent joblessness, and learning how to talk to the ceiling with my back on a couch, I finally blurted out, "I stick my finger down my throat three times a day and throw up. I've been throwing up for years. I'm bulimic. Okay? I have no intention of stopping. Ever. Why would I? I don't want to. Get it? I'm not stopping. That's it. End of discussion. And nothing you say will ever convince me to change. I hope we're clear on this. We're clear, Dr. Landau, right? Right! Okay!!"

Six months later I stopped. One morning I went to the freezer and didn't open a half gallon of rocky road ice cream. I don't know why. I know one thing though: All those disjointed words and half sentences, all those complaining, awkward phrases shaping incomplete monologues blurted out to a sixty-five-year-old woman smoking a cigarette for fifty minutes five times a week, made the difference. It was the talking cure; the talking cure that gave me a way out of addiction; the damn talking cure.

Secrets

I used to think of myself as an attractive victim, a sort of sweet, misunderstood casualty. No one mistook me for the fat woman in the freak show. But I was. And I got away with it. I became a master, as well as a fraud. My secret, with all the little secrets it spawned, encouraged a broad spectrum of subterfuge. I lied to myself, and I kept lying. I never owned up to the truth of bulimia's predatory nature. Yet I gave five years of my life to a ravenous hunger that had to be filled at any expense. I lived under the shadow of isolation in a self-made prison of secrets and lies.

In a culture where confession is a means to broader economic horizons, coming clean at such a late date is not only suspect but anticlimactic. I wish I'd been brave enough to tell Mom before she became entrenched in the uncertainty of Alzheimer's. I told my sisters recently. Dorrie was sympathetic, and Robin remembered I ate a lot of hamburgers back in the day, but neither had much curiosity. Who cares thirty years after the fact? Nobody, really. The thought of becoming number—what?—seventy-five on a "Famous Bulimics" list is like aspiring to footnote status in a file labeled "Eating Disorders." Why bother? I guess partly because confession is at the very least an admission of guilt and partly because there's a humbling aspect to recognizing footnote status. I know "coming clean" is not going to deliver the flattering picture I prefer to roll out with great effort year after year. I don't expect sympathy. I don't expect commiseration. I don't expect to be understood. What I expect is to be released from the burden of hiding.

Maybe

The miracle of getting over bulimia is almost as strange as being its slave. Nothing remains of my former craving. If anything, I have a borderline mistrust for the whole process of consumption. I haven't touched meat in twenty-five years. I'm not remotely drawn to the preparation of food. I'm not hungry. I've had it all, and I've had enough. When I was a bulimic, constantly balancing the extremes of impulsivity and control was sort of like performing. After I stopped throwing up, acting—my lifelong chosen profession—came back into the picture. I started to study with Marilyn Fried, who helped me rediscover the world of expressed feelings. My commitment became more intense than it was when I was too young and too fucked up to take advantage of the opportunity I was given at the Neighborhood Playhouse.

Sandy Meisner used to make arcane pronouncements about how much better our acting would be when we got older and had more experience. Now that I'm the age he was when he stressed the necessity of being more mature in order to become a fully realized actor, now that life has become so much more engaging, if unfathomable, it's hard to believe the accumulated knowledge I'm ready to give isn't what audiences are always interested in. I guess life is always throwing curveballs. Like bulimia, acting is a paradox. Unlike bulimia, acting is a wild ride, shared in the company of other actors. Even though "living truthfully in the given imaginary moment" is not always what you had in mind, it's always a great adventure.

These days I'm trying to learn to listen with the hunger I once reserved for my obsession. The talking cure saved me, it's true, but listening may help me become part of a community. Maybe becoming one of many by doing something as simple as adding my name to a list of bulimics—famous, not so famous, and not famous at all—will give me the courage to cross a threshold that could transform me into the kind of Atticus Finch–type person I always wished I could be. Maybe. Anything's better than the self-imposed loneliness I endured in secret.

Here's to the names, all the names, on that long, long, long, long, long list of ordinary women: names like Carolyn Jennings, Stephanie Armstrong, Allison Kreiger Walsh, Kristen Moeller, Lori Henry, Margie Hodgin, Gail Schoenbach, Sharon Pikus, and now Diane Keaton Hall.

6

THE UPHILL CLIMB
VERSUS THE DOWNHILL SLIDE

Grin and Bare It

There was my career. There was Woody. There was Dr. Landau. There was the record of my dreams. There were my obtuse journals with the list of quotations punctuating my concerns. "I used to worry about being like this. Not knowing more. But now, now, I don't worry anymore." (Sixty-year-old Coney Island resident) "Please stand a little closer apart." (Michael Curtiz) "You see someone on the street and essentially what you notice about them is the flaw." (Diane Arbus) "I wanted to be many things and greatness besides. It was a hopeless task. I never managed to learn to really love another person; only to make the sound of it." (A suicide note) "Look, you don't have that much time." (Walker Evans)

In New York I started making collages again. There was the series called "Grin and Bare It," with pictures of rotting teeth overlaid with captions like "I never knew teeth could be so interesting" or "This middle-aged patient was presented at the oral surgery clinic with the most pronounced case of black hairy tongue ever examined at our institution" or "Hutchinson's Teeth is thought to be an oral manifestation of congenital syphilis." There was the black sketchbook I called "Death Notices." On each page I cut out a photograph of a person from a magazine, erased their face, stamped "Death Notices" across the surface, and glued a random name underneath. Whew!! Finally there was a spate of little notebooks illustrated with sentences from vintage books I bought at the 26th Street flea market. "I am raving." "Hurt, hurt, hurt, hurt, hurt." "Who am I?" "We all die." "The vicious Cycle of Obesity." "'Don't,' she said, holding her ground. 'Don't do that.'" What can I say except it's all too true.

Most of my creative endeavors were nothing more than glorified basket-weaving, another form of insurance against a relapse with a two-pound box of See's Candies peanut brittle. I don't think my artistic solutions to psychological problems were the same as Mom's collage work, journals, and photography. I was lucky because I was young and had more outlets to help overcome my struggles or, at the very least, live with what Dr. Landau termed "anxiety neurosis." On the West Coast, Mom was sailing into the wind alone.

Every cultural experience came to me by way of Woody Allen, my boyfriend. He took me to the movies, where we saw Ingmar Bergman's *Persona* and Luis Buñuel's *The Dis-*

creet *Charm of the Bourgeoisie.* On Madison Avenue we looked in the windows of Serge Sabarsky's gallery of German expressionist paintings. We walked to the Museum of Modern Art and saw the Diane Arbus exhibition curated by John Szarkowski. I took a class in drawing and silk screening. I learned to print my photographs. With Dr. Landau, I examined Then versus Now and Now because of Then. She introduced Freud's "penis envy." Feminists claimed it labeled women as failed men. We took to discussing envy. It turned out I had a fair share of green to examine before I could understand many of my emotional shortcomings.

I still longed for a mother's guidance and found an ideal substitute in Landau. She wasn't the charmed listener Mom was. We didn't hang out at the kitchen counter and share laughs. But she made all the difference. There was no hand-holding as she tried to hammer in the futility of distorting fantasy into reality by quietly paying attention to my steady stream of talk.

Landau knew the world was populated with OTHERS, not just Diane Hall of Orange County. She was a great rep for all the people in my life. Her goal was to help me come to terms with my grandiose expectations. Landau's theory that reality was more exciting than fantasies went in one ear and out the other. Choosing the freedom to be uninteresting never quite worked for me. As much as she tried, and she tried hard, I never found a home in the arms of a man either.

I finally moved out of the 82nd Street studio with its bathtub in the kitchen and found a new apartment at 73rd and Third. Being three thousand miles away from Mom helped me deny any guilt I had over abandoning her. I was in a new business, the business of battling my self-inflicted wounds with activities that kept me away from the toilet down the hall. But more than anything there was . . .

My Career

In 1971 I was cast in Efrem Zimbalist Jr.'s series *The F.B.I.* Here's what I remember. Nothing—except the producers checked my background before I was hired, to make sure I wasn't a criminal.

I also got a guest-starring role in Mike Connors's big hit series *Mannix*. My first shot from the episode named "The Color of Murder" was a two-page monologue. As a gun-toting murderess, I had to scream and yell my way down the middle of a huge warehouse with nothing to hold on to until I broke down and confessed. Terrified, I burst into tears and asked to be let go. "Touch" Connors, as he was affectionately referred to from his old days of playing basketball at UCLA with coach John Wooden, asked everyone to leave the set and walked me through the scene as many times as I needed. I fell in love with him. Not every big star is kind enough to take the time with a frightened young actress. Touch is still hanging in at eighty-six with his bride of more than fifty years, Mary Lou.

In 1972 there was my big break—or so I thought—with the movie of *Play It Again, Sam*. Susan Anspach, who starred opposite Jack Nicholson in *Five Easy Pieces,* joined the cast. I was fascinated by her mysterious manner, until the day she came up to me and told me to stop smiling so much. It would create more laugh lines.

Here's what I can't forget about the first *Godfather:* Dick Smith, the Academy Award–winning makeup artist; and Al Pacino. It was Dick Smith's idea to stick a ten-pound blond wig on my head, where it sat throughout the entire movie like a ton of bricks. I hated that wig almost as much as the red lipstick and starched broad-shouldered suits Theadora Van Runkle designed from the period. I didn't have a clue why I was cast as an elegant WASP. I'm convinced I would have been let go if it weren't for the fact that Paramount begged Francis Ford Coppola to fire Al, until they were blown away by the rushes of Michael Corleone's assassination of Captain McCluskey. Somehow I managed to slip under the radar. It wouldn't have made that much difference if I was replaced or not. I was just a blond-wigged WASP in the Godfather's world.

I met Al Pacino at O'Neals' bar near Lincoln Center. He had been named the Most Promising New Broadway Star in the critically acclaimed *Does a Tiger Wear a Necktie?* We were told to get to know each other before we auditioned for *The Godfather.* I was nervous. The first thing I noticed about Al was his nose. It was long like a cucumber. The second thing I noticed was the kinetic way he moved. He seemed nervous too. I don't remember talking about the script. I remember his killer Roman nose sitting in the middle of what remains a remarkable face. It was too bad he wasn't available, but neither was I. Even so, for the next twenty years Al Pacino would be my only recurring "unattainable great."

In 1973 Woody Allen directed me for the first time. It was *Sleeper,* and it was a piece of cake until the day Woody decided he wasn't happy with a scene we were about to shoot. He went into his trailer and came out a half hour later with a new script. His character had become Blanche DuBois from *A Streetcar Named Desire* and mine was Marlon Brando's Stanley Kowalski. Marlon Brando? Besides being introduced to Mr. Brando at the reading of *The Godfather,* the only encounter we shared was when he passed me on the set and said, "Nice tits." That wasn't going to help. Then I remembered *On the Waterfront* and the line "I coulda been a contender. I coulda been somebody, instead of a bum, which is what I am." I repeated it over and over and over before starting to memorize the lines. In the end Woody and I performed our *Streetcar* parody. But the memory of Terry Malloy's "I coulda been somebody, instead of a bum, which is what I am" is what remains.

Then There Was *The Godfather: Part II*

I was scared as I waited for Francis and Al to rehearse what I now refer to as the "It was an abortion" scene. I told myself I didn't care about *The Godfather* or Al Pacino, but I did. Especially about Al Pacino. He was going with Tuesday Weld. Jill Clayburgh was out, or hovering, like so many others. Things had skyrocketed for Al. He had become an iconic, larger-than-life figure on billboards all over town. He was Michael Corleone. He was Serpico. At the time of the rehearsal we weren't speaking, or, rather, he wasn't speaking to me. Maybe I said something to hurt his feelings, I don't remember. In any event, before our supposed altercation, I managed to worm my way into his good graces by teaching him how to drive in the parking lot of the Cal Neva Hotel in Lake Tahoe.

Al was uncomfortable with the location of the brakes, and he couldn't comprehend the difference between the left- and the right-hand blinking signals. Worse, and far more dangerous, he kept his foot on the gas pedal no matter how many times I told him to press the brake if he wanted to stop. This made for a lot of laughs but a very uncertain ride. In some ways Al reminded me of Randy: He was so sensitive that he was insensitive to his surroundings. I know that sounds like an odd description for the Godfather, but sometimes I swear Al must have been raised by wolves. There were normal things he had no acquaintance with, like the whole idea of enjoying a meal in the company of others. He was more at home eating alone standing up. He did not relate to tables or the conversations people had at them.

We rehearsed the scene as if everything was fine. When Francis got around to shooting it, every take felt completely unexpected, especially Michael Corleone's slap. That was one of the most compelling things about *The Godfather:* the appearance of formality that masked the raw violence exploding in scene after scene. Recently I went to a screening and fell in love with Al all over again. The whole package. You know what I came away with? It was better he'd been raised by wolves. It was better he couldn't drive. It was better he didn't love me and got mad without an explanation. It was worth it, all of it, just to be in that scene with him, just to feel his face against mine. I was Kay, in a role I never related to yet gave me what little I know of Al Pacino. For me the *Godfather*s, all three of them, were about one thing—Al. It was as simple as that. As for the role of Kay? What epitomized it? The picture of a woman standing in a hallway waiting for permission to be seen by her husband.

Journal Entry—Dick Smith, 1974

It's early. They put me in room 404 at the Sheraton in downtown Los Angeles across the street from MacArthur Park. I have a view. I like the room. It has bay windows. Below I can see people come and go; Francis in his limo, Dean Tavoularis in his Mercedes. Only blocks away twenty-four people were killed in a fire last Friday.

I'm sick about the scene. Francis will be up soon. I'm scared. Dick Smith has his makeup brush close to my face. I know I have to stop writing. He insists the actors sit still in the makeup chair. I wonder if he was like this with Marlon Brando. I can smell an orange being eaten by his assistant. I see steam from the water boiling in a pot.

Dick Smith, 2011

Belmont Village, a retirement residence in Burbank, is home to ladies who dine at five-thirty, at least a dozen heroes from World War II, a few youngsters in their sixties, a host of elderly men and women struggling in their late eighties, and now the artist and poet, my brother, John Randolph Hall. On the door to Randy's one-bedroom apartment is a sign: PLEASE DO NOT ENTER. I'M LEARNING HOW TO THINK. And he is.

Every Saturday Randy and I walk to Foster's Freeze for a soft vanilla cone. And every Saturday we see Dick Smith sitting in one of the chairs that line the back of the lobby. Dick Smith, the Academy Award–winning makeup artist, lives at Belmont Village too. Last week Randy's knit cap was pulled low. Mine, a bowler, hit the rim of my glasses. As we got on the elevator, so did Dick Smith. I knew he didn't like hats, but when he said, "Take that hat off," I said, "Thank you, Dick, but I'm keeping it on." That was when he reached over and grabbed Randy's hat off his head.

Dick never liked hats. It's hard to understand. But then, it's hard to understand why Gordon Willis, the cinematographer of all three *Godfather*s, hated makeup artists like Dick Smith. Make no mistake about it—Dick Smith hated Gordon Willis too. It could be that Randy and I, hidden underneath the security of our hats, brought back his resentment of Gordon Willis, or even of Marlon Brando, the jokester. Maybe Dick Smith's award-winning prosthetic makeup had been ruined one too many times by Mr. Brando's notorious antics or the gray fedora he wore when Don Vito Corleone died in his tomato garden.

All I know is, Dick Smith is back and he still hates hats. Marlon Brando came back too. Nine years ago I was walking down a hall at the UCLA Medical Center when I saw him shuffle toward me as he held on to a companion. There was no "Nice tits" this time. He looked at me blank-faced. Dick

Smith, in the early stages of Alzheimer's disease, looks at me every Saturday. What does he see? An inappropriate woman with an equally inappropriate man walking through the lobby of his home, wearing hats? I know what I see—a home inhabited by a host of unique individuals who will in all likelihood soon enough become part of what Duke refers to as the Sea of White Crosses.

Love and Death

Throughout the filming of *Love and Death*, Woody wrote to me. I was his endearing oaf. He was my "White Thing." Although his body was fit and well proportioned, he treated it like it was a strange assortment of disembodied appendages. His feet never touched the ground. He was constantly in the care of one doctor or another. We were quite a couple, one more hidden than the other. We both wore hats in public, and he always held my hand or, rather, gripped it without letting go. People were to be avoided. I had him pegged as a cross between a "White Thing" and the cockroach you couldn't kill. We shared a love of torturing each other with our failures. He could sling out the insults, but so could I. We thrived on demeaning each other. His insights into my character were dead on and—duh!—hilarious. This bond remains the core of our friendship and, for me, love.

> Greetings Worm,
>   We have enough rehearsal time, but not as much as in L.A. Still, I think Love and Death will be easier than

Sleeper as there is not a lot of . . . falls and spills and water stunts . . . Our dialogue exchanges should be brisk and lively . . . but we'll get into that . . . so snookums . . . speak with you soon.

Also finished 1st draft of 2 New Yorker pieces. Hey! My book—Getting Even—is a hit in France. Go figure. You remain a flower—too, too delicate for this harsh world & Dorrie is a flower & your mother is a flower & your father a vegetable & Randy is a flower in his way & Robin is a cat. And I remain a weed.—Will call.

Woody

Greetings Worm,

I am jettisoning some old socks in my travel bag to make room for some idiot's sunflower seeds. Guess who? You, my pal, are my cross to bear.

So they're all saying I'm a genius—but you know better, you little hellgrammite. Are you sure they're not calling me the "White Thing?" "And he changes his underwear to sleep in." And all the things you call me rather than genius? I am tortured with the most incredible dreams of sexuality that revolve around you and a large 2E BRA that speaks Russian.

That genial wit and good egg, Woody

Lamp-head,-simpleton-oaf—

I have decided to let your family make me rich! It turns out they are wonderful material for a film. A quite serious one, although one of the three sisters is a fool and a clown. (I think you can guess which, ducky!) I didn't send you a big letter because you're coming to Paris soon. I wonder if your observations about my family clock them as weirdly as I see yours? Do you have insights into my father & mother? I can imagine. The blind perceiving the blind. Last nite I had a tender dream about me & my mother. First dream of her in years. Wonder why? I wept in the dream & ate my laundry. Just kidding—I ate her boiled chicken which tastes worse.

Love from the fabulous Mister A, a man with healing humour.

Mom and the Downhill Slide, 1975

I'm sitting in the TV room in my blue, white-trimmed robe with my hair in hot rollers so I can go to my one day a week afternoon job looking acceptable. Why am I a compulsive conformist? Why do I always wear a scarf at my neck? Why am I always sprayed down with a controlled hairstyle? Why do my shoes always match my pants? Why do I always flash the stiff, put-on smile for passersby? Why do I do this? I don't know. I feel like I'm under a foot of oppression as I take my last sip of coffee and my last drag off the Parliament cigarette. I don't smoke. Why am I doing this?

Last night was the start of a continuing awkward and permanent silence. Damn it, I have such waves of insecurity. I'm no one to anyone. People look at me and see a

midlife woman on the downhill slide. 55 is approaching.
My brain is getting thinner. If there's one thing I don't want
to lose, it's my ability to think. I feel old and intolerant. It's
like I'm shutting the world out. I don't like it. I really must
not drink so much alcohol.

It all started Easter Sunday. Jack and I went to Mary's
to help her tackle the ordeal of tax returns, which she had
refused to pay. As expected, she opened the door and
started in on the Damn Government. It took Jack hours of
pain & anguish while Mary stood over him justifying her
refusal to file a California tax return, even though she'd re-
ceived several notices about past discrepancies. Jack warned
her repeatedly that she'd been playing with fire. Mary
wouldn't listen. "Let them come to the door. I don't care.
I'll just play dumb. That's what I'll do. I'm not afraid." Jack
almost lost it. "Goddamn it, Mother, just let me get on with
this. I'm tired & I don't want any more crap."

I brought a pot roast, but all she did was complain
about that too. Iowa is the only place with tender beef. And
as for food in Los Angeles. Forget it. Only cafeteria style
tastes any good at all. Then she started in on Randy and his
poems. "What do his poems mean anyway; who ever heard
of writing about celery? It ain't a poem you can under-
stand, like Roses are Red. I don't know what he's talking
about. I don't get it." And then as if to torture me she kept
going on, "What exactly does Robin do besides take care of
people who are dying?" And, "Does Dorrie like that Peter
guy? What nationality is he anyway?" And, "What about
that Diane, flying all the way back to N.Y. before Easter?
Doesn't she want to be at home? I guess she hates flying,

huh? Touch of Jack showing there. Oh well, it's a weird old world." And . . . And . . . And. All I thought was, What happened? We used to do family things on Easter. I'd make brand-new outfits for all the kids. We'd go to church. I'd cook. We'd all be together, Dorrie, Randy, Robin, and Diane . . . all of us together. So many things have changed. When I think back on my four children, I remember each little warm body meant something to me I could never put into words; never.

When we got home Dorrie called to say she wasn't coming down. I tried to read, but couldn't get Dorrie out of my thoughts. Why doesn't she come see ME? I tried to rub the thoughts out. I started to think of actions I wanted to take, but rationalized I shouldn't. I kept thinking if I'm so miserably maladjusted to this life, my absence would only be felt for a short time. And anyway, my responsibilities with the family are over. They no longer look to me for guidance. It's more like I'm the one they're stuck being responsible for. My company isn't sought after. Whatever I have allowed to happen has also brought on this horrible lack of confidence. I'm intimidated. I have no one to tell my concerns to, NO ONE. I've let myself come to a very sad state, not only sad, but stagnant. I try to talk to Jack but I can't. He doesn't care. He doesn't want to LISTEN.

I have a secret longing to set out alone & do what I want to do. Why don't I? It would be better than driving with Jack to the foreclosure auction, like I did last week. The radio kept blaring out the awful news of Idi Amin executing dissenters in Uganda. I asked Jack where the dial on the AM radio was—he kept pointing to the switch button.

"Dial, Dorothy, DIAL." "Don't shout at me!" I said. "I'm NOT shouting at you." Then silence.

We drove past South Coast Plaza Shopping Mall, where the new I. Magnin's is going up near Bullock's. We were silent as we drove past Long Beach, past Downey, past the City of Commerce, and on to Torrance. I saw an overturned truck when we reached the Magnolia off ramp. It didn't register because there was so much anger in me, all I could think about was the fact that I can't live according to Jack's list of rules anymore. I'm sick of being smothered by all the talk of real estate, and taxes, and how to buy, and Money, Money, Money. We passed a Motel 6 sign next to a Lutheran church, next to a Jewish temple, next to a used-car sales lot, where I saw Toyotas, Ford Torino wagons, Chevy Vegas, Pintos and Datsuns, and still we were silent. We passed a man in the driver's seat teasing his hair into a stand-up position. A plane landed at LAX. It was hot. The auction started at 10. I wanted out.

I've created this solitude. I'm drowning in the worst depression I can remember. I've always tried to hide my feelings. Things, even little things, seem to dislodge my frail grip on the handle of positivity. I completely succumb to the dark side. At one time I fought with all I knew to prevent these unwelcome attacks. I did a great deal of pretending. I would say to myself, "I'm not depressed, I'm not—I'm not." I kept covering up, pushing back, denying, in an effort to appear "normal." When the kids were alone with me, I would be attentive, involved, interested, and warm. When Jack got home from work the pretense began—fake actions and words in order to present a calm unruffled atmosphere.

Someone I can't remember once said, "No one gets mad or even raises their voice in your household." What an indictment, but at the time I considered it the achievement of a good mother.

And Finally ...

This will be strange because I am going to be honest. By honest, I mean I won't leave out details like I usually do. I'm sitting in front of the fireplace—a fire is burning; burning one of our dining room chairs. I'm a bit shaky, but I'm not lost, frustrated, erratic, or illogical. The chair has almost burned away. I don't care. Last night all my framed photos were thrown. There's splintered glass everywhere. The flowers Diane sent are all over the floor. The table has a big gouge. I have red bruises on my face. There are black and blue marks on my arms and legs. Where in hell are WE HEADING?

I can't vent like Jack does. This is the key to our mismatch. My anger comes out in cold unbearable behavior. It eats on him until he explodes. I don't know why I constantly practice challenging Jack. It's so out of hand. He says the salad at Coco's is good. I turn quiet, because he didn't say, "But not as good as yours." He asks if I trimmed the bush in the garden and I say, "Why do you want to know?" He asks where I'd like to eat, I say, "I don't know." He says, "Well, how about Dillmans?" I say, "We always go where you want to go." He says, "There's a program on TV that sounds good." I say, "I read it wasn't that great." He says, "What's for dinner?" I say, "You'll like it." He says, "Typical Doro-

thy answer." Then I'm mad all evening. I don't know how
many times I've told myself that nobody really has my wel-
fare in mind but me. My care is in the hands of ME.
  Jack left me a note. "I wish to hell you'd leave me." I
called and told him I wanted to, just as soon as he figured
out how to do it. BULL SHIT. I'm angry. I feel totally mis-
understood. I know things will never get better. When I
think of Jack, something gets ahold of me. I do NOT want
to complain. I WILL NOT—but I WANT better. This is my
right and, in a funny way, my responsibility. I need stimula-
tion. After a life of working and planning for the fam-
ily . . . I need others. My head gets too lost when it's only
me hanging around the house all day, every day. After last
night I thought I would kill myself rather than go through
the torture of losing my mind.

From Diane

Mom, the brain fed you an overload of negative data, which
you held on to for dear life. Why couldn't you stop beating
up yourself or the people around you—i.e., Dad? It must
have been hard to take into consideration what it was like for
him to come from a money-driven, half-crazy, fatherless
home, complete with Mary Alice Hall as Mother. The effect
of such an upbringing did not make Dad an easygoing
liberal-minded kind of guy. Don't think I don't remember
his entrances and how they disrupted the mystique we created with a kind of dreaded reality. Dad was the enemy we
kept close. It wasn't just you, it was all of us.

As the recipient of whatever public validation there was to be gleaned from the business of civil engineering in Orange County, Dad was dynamic. You went a different path. You read Virginia Woolf, who drowned herself in a river, and Anne Sexton, who locked herself in a car and turned on the engine. You had a poet's appreciation of language, a beautiful face, and an irresistibly alluring, almost inhuman amount of charm, but these gifts didn't sustain you. By the time 1975 rolled around, your best friend—your journal—became the only release. Our little gang of five had all but dissolved. You were writing your story, I understand, but, Mom, did it have to be so distressing? When was everything going to get better? When were the positive thoughts written in longhand going to reappear?

If I told you how much I loved the sound of your laughter, would you have taken more pride in who you were? If, way back, I made you understand how proud I was to be the daughter of a "really, really special" former Mrs. Los Angeles, would that have made a difference? If you knew how fast I rushed home from Willard Junior High School the day Dave Garland poked his finger in my padded bra and made fun of me, would you have finally acknowledged you were irreplaceable? If I reminded you of the pleasure it gave me to hang out at the kitchen counter and watch you make your mid-afternoon snack of longhorn cheddar cheese and Wheat Thins, with sweet gherkins on the side, would that have changed anything?

Remember how we used to drive around downtown Santa Ana on Wednesday evenings after Bullock's department store closed? Remember how I sat shotgun checking out possible "finds"? Remember how I snuck out of the car and rummaged through the trash bins to see if there were any treasures to be found? Was it as much fun for you as it was for me? Did you get a kick out of making sure the coast was clear before I shoved that really cool bathroom shelf into the trunk? We thought it was perfect, remember? But then, so were you. You were the perfect find. Could it have been more fun, Mom, driving home in our Buick station wagon back in the early days of suburbia, just us, turning an ordinary afternoon into something extraordinary? Remember how you told me about the new store in La Mirada called Ohrbach's and how we could buy brand names for a fourth of what they cost at Bullock's? Remember the time I was sick over not being invited to join Zeta Tee, the second-best sorority at Santa Ana High School, even though they'd asked Leslie? You told me to have patience. Zeta Tee could wait for later; besides, the girls were a little trashy, weren't they, and didn't the so-called "grooviest" member get pregnant? Then suddenly I'd hear, "Oh, my God, Diane, look. Diane, you've got to see this," or "Di-annie, check this out." I'd look and see an ordinary boy riding a bike past Me-N-Ed's Pizza on McFadden and Bristol. It was nothing, but it was something. It was just an ordinary boy passing by, but somehow it was unforgettable and somehow it tore me away from pressing tragedies like not making the cut with Zeta Tee.

Did you ever pat yourself on the back for your greatest gift, just being you? I'm sorry the small rewards weren't enough. I understand great expectations. Oh, Mom, Mom, you were such a game gal in so many ways. I wish I could have made the disappointment of your unfulfilled longings magically disappear with the memory of our Wednesday evening adventures, now lost in time.

Did all that writing in all those journals make it worse? Did it exacerbate your isolation? If only we could re-edit our lives and make a couple of different choices, right, Mom? Where would it have taken us? Now I'm alone, juggling with a memoir that's also your memoir. Would you have approved of my choices? Am I misrepresenting you? I'll never know. I can only hope you would have forgiven me for revealing your demons, but, in my defense, you wrote it so beautifully. You would have wanted me to share it, right? I hope so. I wish it weren't too late to go back to see what you might have felt.

Mind Priorities—April 1975

Day 1. My energy is up. Day 2. My motivation is up. Day 3. My personal drive is up. Day 4. My spiritual growth is high. Day 5. I am on a higher plane. I work at this. Day 6. I am throwing out the undesirable from my system. Day 7. I have reached a HIGH beautiful spiritual level. Day 8. I like ME. Day 9. I do meaningful things—think logically—move with grace and ease. Day 10. I love myself—am beautiful inside and out. Day 11. I am not smothered when Jack is around. Day 12. I can still maintain personal beauty and countenance. Day 13. I show love and feel stable inside. Day 14. I am bigger. Day 15. I am ready to take others' comments, realizing I don't know their intentions or real meaning. Day 16. I am able to bounce back mentally. Day 17. I am positive. Day 18. I contribute to bringing out the very best in people I am around. Day 19. Diane, Randy, Robin, and Dorrie all fall under my mental thought waves. Day 20. Jack is on the same wave too. Day 21. I value my flashes of creative thought. Day 22. I displace negative thoughts completely and respond to events accordingly. Day 23. I am proud of my spiritual being and the growth I have in this area. Day 24. I believe my spirituality softens the harshness of reality. Day 25. I am thin, one hundred and thirty-five pounds. Day 26. I am passing through the midlife mess and making it. Day 27. I am wise to the needs of others. Day 28. I am continually gaining knowledge. Day 29. I am the beneficiary of all that I surround myself with. Day 30. I am enriching my environment in every way I know. Day 31. I am developing my mind and using it in my continuing search for knowledge.

Days of the Week

Sunday the 2nd—BE HEALTHY
Monday the 3rd—GET THIN
Tuesday the 4th—SELL COLLINS ISLAND HOUSE
Wednesday the 5th—MOVE TO NEAT PLACE
Thursday the 6th—MAKE NEW FRIENDS
Friday the 7th—CULTIVATE OLD ONES
Saturday the 8th—TRAVEL
Sunday the 9th—MENTALLY GROW—EXPAND
Monday the 10th—TAKE MORE CARE WITH—
Tuesday the 11th—COOKING
Wednesday the 12th—BE LESS CONCERNED—
Thursday the 13th—WITH MYSELF

Friday the 14th—BE LIGHTER ABOUT THINGS
Saturday the 15th—LAUGH A LOT
Sunday the 16th—TALK MORE

Dorothy-isms

After the downhill slide, and living under the influence of Jack Hall's "power of positive thinking," Dorothy created her own catalog of cheerful bromides to combat depression. The itemized series of pep talks and wishful pick-me-ups had a function: to make her feel better. This year was going to be different. It was the year of Dorothy's "Days of the Week" and "What I Am Thankful For." Itemizing catchphrases as if they were wishes that would come true was like praying to a benevolent God who encouraged repetition as a means to an end—a cheerful one. Mother organized information and kept track of changes by classifying her adages chronologically or grouping them by theme. She did not resort to the unsorted or miscellaneous. All homilies worthy of inclusion were gathered together with some criteria in mind.

She did not pass on her Pollyanna-isms, or make reference to her Mount Whitney of words, to anyone. I suspect she shielded us from her "healing business" because somewhere deep down she knew her remedies were best left unexamined. For example, once having written "I am enriching my environment in every way I know," Mother avoided analyzing it. Why would she? She was smart. She knew she was a harsh critic. She knew she would have been disappointed in the results. Mother's list of platitudes rose higher and higher, all the way to the top of the biggest list of all, the "Forgotten List." Once she forgot an idea, Mother was free to rediscover it as if it was forever and always the first "I-am-ism" on the first day of the first week of the first month of the year 1975.

Bogged down by the same dilemmas, Mom and I shared a fear of failure, a concern for what others think, demeaning comparisons, and low self-esteem. In a way, Dorothy's bromides were a healthier version of my throwing up. After she "did her business," her system was purged and, like me, she felt better until she needed a new resolution to help cope with getting through yet another day. As a little girl, Mom put two and two together after she saw her friend Jean Cutler write "I will not put gum under my desk" on the blackboard one hundred times. Dorothy saved her one hundred "I will have more self-confidence"s for when she needed it the most—later, much later.

Itemizing what she accomplished or, "doggone it," how she was going to appreciate herself for once did help her weather the storm. I just wonder if it would have been different with an audience. As her only congregation, Mom was always in the business of being her own best friend. It's true Mother's put-ups gave her a much needed break—they helped smooth out the bumpy road—but they didn't prod her to go further. Dorothy, the good girl, the good mother, but not always the good wife, had nothing to show for the role she accepted. Instead there was the day the truck came with the furniture. The day she got rid of the old couch for the new Pottery Barn linen love seats. The day she planted geraniums outside the picture window. And all those well-intended slogans on paper. There was that. And that was it. Nothing more, and no one to share it with, except Jack.

On the Other Side of the Same Coin

Mother made her big choice early. She married. I made mine late. I adopted. At fifty-four Dorothy was put out to pasture with thirty-two more years of living staring her in the face. At sixty-five there is no pasture, and I'm not lonely. With an all-consuming new occupation—parenthood—and an extended family, I'm busy. Eleven years older than Dorothy when she quietly penciled in her parade of panaceas, I'm running around like a chicken with its head cut off, but I like it. I love it. It's hard to imagine life without Dexter's phone issues and Duke's preadolescent poop jokes, which he insists on sharing as I drive him home from swim practice every day. We sing along to Katy Perry's new song, "Firework." We think it's really funny when he hits my arm every time he spots a VW punch buggy. Dexter and Duke have changed my life. People say they're lucky to have me. I don't know about that. That's not the real story. The real story is, I'm the lucky one. They've saved me, and I know what from: myself. Odd, isn't it? My life today is as full as Mother's was when she happily worked overtime raising a growing family in her mid-twenties.

In 2001 A.D. (After Duke), I began my first and only list. It's not that I wanted to. It's that I had to, and when I did, I knew what to call it: "To Do!" In the flurry of life I couldn't afford to have anything, or anybody, overlooked. I couldn't drop the ball. I didn't have time to look for a way to feel better. I had "To Do" it.

To Do! November 2010

1.   The California sign is slated to be finished on Tuesday. The question is, will it fit the brick wall of the Lloyd Wright house? The letters are 5 feet high! Did anybody speak to the neighbors about the trash cans? Who's going to tell Stephanie B. the cabbage plant has to be removed? Let's face it; it's too English for a sustainable native California landscape. And those black plants. Oh my God, they look cruel within the context of the rest of the garden. I know, I know, yet another bad idea.

2.   I've got to turn in the chapter on 1969 . . . as soon as possible.

3.   Call Bill Robinson. I miss him, and Johnny, and little Baby Dylan. I don't know how to keep close to them. Bill was a pivotal factor in the adoption of Dexter, and now that he and Johnny have adopted Dylan he's gone. New York seems so far away. I've got to call him. Do you have any ideas?

4.   When is the *T Magazine* article out?

5.   How about hiring Dorrie to scout out Navajo pictorial blankets? She knows the dealers better than anyone.

6.   I don't know how I dropped the ball on Westmark School's Get Ready for 9th Grade assembly. I have to go.

Should I take the 405 or Mulholland? Anyway, it starts at 2 o'clock. We'll discuss.

7.   Stephanie, you've got to tell me the truth—how many flights do we have to take for the Unique Lives Lecture Series Tour? Who can I rehearse my speech to besides Jessica Kovacevic, who's already been tortured one too many times? I'm starting to get nervous. Speaking of nervous, I don't think I can keep trying to memorize my speech while jogging on the streets of Beverly Hills. The Starline Bus Tours unfailingly drive by while I'm in the middle of rehearsing the final section—you know, when I sing a bit of "Seems Like Old Times." It's awful. I feel like an idiot. Is this speech going to work? Be honest. There's something inherently wrong about addressing my female contemporaries on the subject of me. It's too much. It reminds me of Katharine Hepburn's autobiography, *Me.*

8.   Duke made a Nespresso for Jimmy, the car washer, yesterday. By the way, he's back from the hospital. You'll never believe this; he told me hiccups were the only symptom he had before his gallbladder was removed. Anyway, he wants a sponsorship for his bowling team. What do you think? I say yes. Most important, Duke was proud of himself for, number 1, making the coffee and, number 2, appearing to be generous.

9.   Starting Tuesday, I drive Dexter to swim practice at 4:45 a.m. This means I can sit in the backseat of my mobile office and work on the rewrite of the memoir. I'm way behind.

What to do? At least I'll get in a full two hours without interruptions. Starbucks opens at 5. I'll need it.

As for Dorothy

I am thankful for the beautiful, round full moon last night.
I am thankful for the weekend Jack & I just had in Ojai.
I am thankful for the good feelings I have all at once for no reason.
I am thankful for the friends who respond to me.
I am thankful for my work at Hunter's Bookstore.
I am thankful for my new independence with money.
I am thankful for my more orderly, clear mind.
I take pride in being me, Dorothy D. Hall.

Loving Jack

Number 1. Seeing him is beautiful.
Number 2. We both realize how important we are to one another.
Number 3. The other evening we looked at one another, held hands, and communicated our feelings of love and need.

7

DI-ANNIE HALL

Wake-Up Call, 2009

Getting up at three-thirty A.M. to catch a flight to L.A. after spending six weeks in New York shooting *Morning Glory* doesn't help the vertigo. As I spin my way to the Nespresso machine, waiting for the crystals in my ear to readjust, I think of that first shot on the first day. One minute I was on a mat in a fat suit, playing with a four-hundred-pound sumo wrestler; the next I was on a gurney, in a neck brace, looking up at the machine taking pictures of my brain. Like Humpty Dumpty, I took a great fall.

I think of the nurses at Columbia Presbyterian checking every three hours to see if I was alive. I think of the fall that took Natasha Richardson's life and know I'm lucky. I think of Duke, who said, "Mom, did you lose your memories?" I think of the people I worked with. There was Roger Michell, our bear of a director; beautiful Rachel McAdams; and legendary Harrison Ford. I think of the $65 million he made in 2008, beating out Johnny Depp for the title of number-one box-office winner; that's pretty good for a sixty-five-year-old man. That's a lot of money. I think about money and worry like Dad used to. I worry about Emmie, our seven-year-old shit-eating dog. I worry about Randy's liver, and Robin's daughter, Riley, with her new baby, Dylan. I worry about Duke's lack of boundaries. I worry about Dorrie's antiques business and Dexter's teen years. But mainly I worry about how long I can keep it all going. Which, of course, makes me think of the Unique Lives Lecture Series Tour, where I found myself on the road in Minneapolis, Des Moines, Boston, Toronto, Montreal, and Denver, in Carrie Underwood's new tour bus. What about all those women, my contemporaries, my sisters, in all those auditoriums listening to Diane Keaton—that's me—give a Unique Lecture on the subject of being a woman over sixty? When Stephanie Heaton (not to be confused with Keaton) and I spent the night in Carrie's bus, we pulled over to grab a Starbucks at the World's Largest Truck Stop, and I thought, Okay, I'm no Harrison Ford, but I'm making my way, and it's never boring.

As I wheel my suitcase into the hallway, I start to think about what's waiting for me back in L.A. Oh, God, school again. Already? Duke in third grade, Dex in eighth. Not possible. I think about the restoration of the Wright house I bought before the recession hit. I think about the complications of selling Mom and Dad's two oceanfront homes after the seawall collapsed down the block. I think about Dorrie, who doesn't want to sell; Robin, who does; and Randy, who's oblivious.

I throw on some Diane's Tuberose lipstick by L'Oreal. I think about walking barefoot in Central Park at nine P.M. last night, looking at fireflies while Duke and Dexter laughed themselves down the stainless-steel slide. Will this be the last year Dex allows herself to play like a kid? I think about Duke dressed up in a box seat, watching Billy Elliot tap-dance his way across the Broadway stage. It makes me wish I could live in New York again. I think about waiting in line on Fifth Avenue outside Abercrombie & Fitch with Dex, as she dreamed of boys, and suntans, and love, and kisses. I think about the morning we rode bikes over the Brooklyn Bridge, one of our country's greatest engineering feats in the greatest city of them all. I think of the 59th Street Bridge in *Manhattan* and the block of brownstones Woody and I walked past in the East 70s from *Annie Hall*. I don't want to leave this city. I want to stay. I want to go back to another day, not unlike today, where I also found myself up at three-thirty A.M., only then I was waiting to be picked up for my first day of shooting the Untitled Woody Allen Project in the spring of 1976.

Annie Hall

ALVY: You want a lift?
ANNIE: Oh, why? Uh, you got a car?
ALVY: No, um . . . I was going to take a cab.
ANNIE: Oh, no. I have a car.

ALVY: You have a car? I don't understand why . . . If you have a car, so then why did you say, "Do you have a car?" like you wanted a lift?

ANNIE: I don't, I don't, geez, I don't know. I wasn't . . . I got this VW out there. (To herself) What a jerk, yeah. (To Alvy) Would you like a lift?

ALVY: Sure. Which way you goin'?

ANNIE: Me? Oh, downtown.

ALVY: Down . . . I'm going uptown.

ANNIE: Oh, well, you know, I'm going uptown too.

ALVY: You just said you were going downtown.

ANNIE: Yeah, well, but I can . . .

Make Work Play

Filming *Annie Hall* was effortless. During breaks, Woody would carry around a pack of Camels, take one out of his shirt pocket à la George Raft, flip it into his mouth, blow smoke rings, and never inhale. No one had any serious expectations. We were just having a good time moving through New York's landmark locations. As always, Woody concerned himself with worries about the script. Was it too much like an episode of *The Mary Tyler Moore Show*? I told him he was nuts. Relax.

If a scene wasn't working, Woody would do what he always did: rewrite it while Gordon Willis was setting up the shot. Rewrite frequently meant re-edit. Woody didn't hold his words in high regard; as a result, there was no excess fat in *Annie Hall*. The choice of Gordon Willis as cinematographer was a turning point and an unerring example of Woody breaking the rules. Like many funny men, he had a borderline contempt for comedy. But, unlike others, he used that attitude to invent a host of witty visual approaches that gave *Annie Hall* weight. With Gordon at his side, Woody stopped being afraid of the dark. He learned how to shoot split screens and flashbacks with style. Gordon helped teach him to choreograph the master shot so it could be used to deliver the variety and impact an audience needed without cutting to close-ups. These innovations were new for comedy. *Annie Hall,* all dressed up in shadow and light, moving through time without a lot of arbitrary coverage, was seamless.

Woody's direction was the same. Loosen up the dialogue. Forget the marks. Move around like a real person. Don't make too much of the words, and wear what you want to wear. Wear what you want to wear? That was a first. So I did what Woody said: I wore what I wanted to wear, or, rather, I stole what I wanted to wear from cool-looking women on the streets of New York. Annie's khaki pants, vest, and tie came from them. I stole the hat from Aurore Clément, Dean Tavoularis's future wife, who showed up on the set of *The Godfather: Part II* one day wearing a man's slouchy bolero pulled down low over her forehead. Aurore's hat put the finishing touch on the so-called Annie Hall look. Aurore had style, but so did all the street-chic women livening up SoHo in the mid-seventies. They were the real costume designers of *Annie Hall*.

Well, that's not entirely true. Woody was. Every idea, every choice, every decision, came from the mind of Woody Allen.

A Screening, March 27, 1977

Jack and I held hands at the screening of Annie Hall. *It was closing night of the Filmex Festival in Century City. The theater was flooded with lights and fireworks overhead. Inside, we found seats in the front row only. We chose to sit on the steps at the back of the room.* ANNIE HALL. *I only saw Diane, her mannerisms, expressions, dress, hair, etc., the total her. The story took second place. When she sang, "It Had to Be You" in a room full of talk and confusion, I fought back tears. But the song "Seems Like Old Times" was the hard one to take; so tender. I was exploding inside. I tried to hold it all back. She looked beautiful. Gordon Willis did a very great job on the photography. She chose her own clothes and the gray T-shirt and baggy pants were "down home" for sure.* Annie Hall *is a love story. It seemed real. Annie's camera in hand, her gum chewing, her lack of confidence; pure Diane. The story was tender, funny, and sad. It ended in separation, just like real life.*

The Hall family was comic relief, especially the Randy character, named Duane. Woody's character couldn't understand Duane's unique problems. Colleen Dewhurst as me was not a high spot. The Grammy Hall character was nothing more than a visual gag. And Jack's part was not impressive. The audience loved it though. They were clapping and laughing the whole way through. This will be a very popular movie.

Mom and I never discussed the Hall family as depicted in *Annie Hall*. What was there to discuss? I hadn't seen the movie. When I won the New York Film Critics Circle Award, I figured I'd better get myself to a movie theater before I gave my acceptance speech. It was 1978. I went to a matinee on 59th and Third. There was a smattering of people in the theater. I didn't hear any laughs. Like Mom, I was so consumed by the "me" of it all that I couldn't pay attention to the story. I kept thinking, What's all the fuss about? Predictably, I hated my face, the sound of my voice, and my awful "mannerisms." On the positive side, I knew I was lucky. And I was grateful. I didn't bother myself with the Hall family scenes. They were of no concern. First of all, not one character was even remotely identifiable. Weird Duane, played by Chris Walken, was hilarious but from the planet Mars. Woody's version of my family was comic relief. He wrote a generic WASP family and built some jokes around the dinner table. I didn't give the scene a second thought.

Most people assumed *Annie Hall* was the story of our relationship. My last name is Hall. Woody and I did share a significant romance, according to me, anyway. I did want to be a singer. I was insecure, and I did grope for words. After thirty-five years, does anybody care? What matters is Woody's body of work. *Annie Hall* was his first love story. Love was the glue that held those witty vignettes together. However bittersweet, the message was clear. Love fades. Woody took a risk; he let the audience feel the sadness of goodbye in a funny movie.

At seventy-five, after making forty-five films in forty-five years, he's the only director who without fail secures financing for his annual film. The deal includes complete control and final cut. It's not that other filmmakers haven't earned the right; it's that, in a business incapable of tolerating failure, Woody has chutzpah. And his movies are budgeted with reality in mind. It's a testimony to his particular brand of genius that he can still cast major movie stars while paying them minimum wage. The enticement? Five actors have received six Academy Awards from appearing in a Woody Allen movie, and ten have received nominations.

In the end it all boils down to words. Woody's words. He's either written or co-written every movie he's directed. Writing is the underpinning, infrastructure, point of departure, reason, and pretext for all of it.

A Phone Call

Even though we broke up two years before we shot *Annie Hall,* I was still Woody's sidekick. I can't explain why we continued to click. Maybe, as with an old couch, we were comfortable with each other. We still enjoyed sitting in "Oldies' Row" at the entrance to Central Park, making observations on the parade of humanity passing by. We still had fun with our "kitchen follies" and we still kept planning future projects, but things had changed. He was suddenly the comic genius. I was suddenly getting more opportunities. I met with Warren Beatty for his movie *Heaven Can Wait* and turned him down to hit the bars as Theresa Dunn in *Looking for Mr. Goodbar.* After *Goodbar* finished shooting, I went back to New York. When Warren called me on Christmas Eve, it wasn't about a job.

And he kept calling. In January of 1978 Warren and I

started hanging out. I told myself it was temporary. I could handle it. Sure, he was smart, lawyer-smart. And, yes, he was still a mind-blowing dream of drop-dead gorgeous. I don't know why I thought I could manage things—well, that's not true, I didn't think at all. I fell. And I kept falling for a long time. He grabbed me from the first moment I saw him in the lobby of the Beverly Wilshire Hotel way back in 1972. I looked up, and in the distance I saw my dream come true in person. I also saw that there wasn't a woman within close proximity he didn't scrutinize, except me. He didn't scrutinize me, not then.

To Die For

Warren turned out to be a far more complex character than I could have imagined when I saw him kiss Natalie Wood in *Splendor in the Grass* at the Broadway Theater in Santa Ana. I was in tenth grade. I'd never seen anything like Warren Beatty. By *thing*, I mean he wasn't real. He was to die for. And Natalie Wood? Well, she was me. I was her. When Bud and Deanie were forced to part, I was devastated. I even wrote Mr. Elia Kazan, the director, inquiring why the parents were so opposed to true love. Could he have changed the ending? What was the big deal about different social classes? He did not respond. It's ironic; a couple of weeks ago I caught a glimpse of *Splendor in the Grass* on TV. There they were again, Bud and Deanie, still tormented, still in love. My own romance with Warren was not destined for the long haul either. For us it wasn't circumstance. It was character. I admit there was a smattering of two different worlds mixed in; after all, Warren was "The Prince of Hollywood" and I was, as my dad called me, Di-annie Oh Hall-ie.

Warren was infamous. We used to gossip about his conquests after Martha Graham dance class at the Neighborhood Playhouse. Cricket Cohen knew a girl who knew a girl he picked up and took back to his hotel room at the Waldorf Astoria. Oh, my God, how awful, how humiliating. We all swore we would never fall into that kind of trap. Not us.

What I didn't know was, once Warren chose to shine his light on you, there was no going back. Within his gaze I was the most captivating person in the world. He fed on every nuance of my lopsided face and saw beauty. It was enchanting, but it was scary too. I was straddling two lives, in two different locations. I was with Warren, but because of *Annie Hall* everyone still thought I was Woody's girl.

Warren opened every door with his bullshit detector fully charged. Always searching for what lay hidden behind the façade, he was the only person who was curious enough to ask me if my Annie Hall glasses were prescription. Nailed. While Woody encouraged my artistic endeavors with things like "P.S. Your new photos arrived. The best yet! Really!" Warren would look askance at one of my collages and say, "You're a movie star. That's what you wanted. You got it. Now deal with it. What is all this art stuff going to get you anyway?" That's what I liked about him; he told it like he saw it. And he saw it with a lot of variables.

When I compare Mother's relationship with Father to mine with Warren, there's no question Warren's promises were far more seductive than Jack Hall's could ever be. After

I confessed how terrified I was to fly, Warren surprised me as I was about to board a flight to New York, took my hand, walked me into the plane, sat down still holding my hand, and never let go until we landed. Once safe on the ground he kissed me, turned around, and flew back to L.A. On Valentine's Day he bought me a sauna for one bathroom and a steam room for the other. He was full of magnanimous gestures. He also filled my head with crazy thoughts: I had enormous potential. I could be a director, a politician, as well as one of the most revered actresses in the world if I wanted. I would laugh and tell him he was out of his mind. But I loved it, every second, and I loved him, especially his insane largesse.

Diane

There was a moment when we first sat down at dinner last night when I looked at you and you seemed to have such an unfair allotment of gifts that it frightened me. Plus you had time on your side too.

You've made a lot of money for the movie business and your percentages for the profits haven't been so huge that you should feel guilty about taking some of the industry's money and making your own film. I think they'd be happy to do it.

Stop messing around and do it. You'd do it better than anybody. You know more than anybody. Its rough edges would be fascinating. I can set it up early. And either produce or get completely out of your way.

Do it now. It will make you feel much better about movies in general and acting in particular.

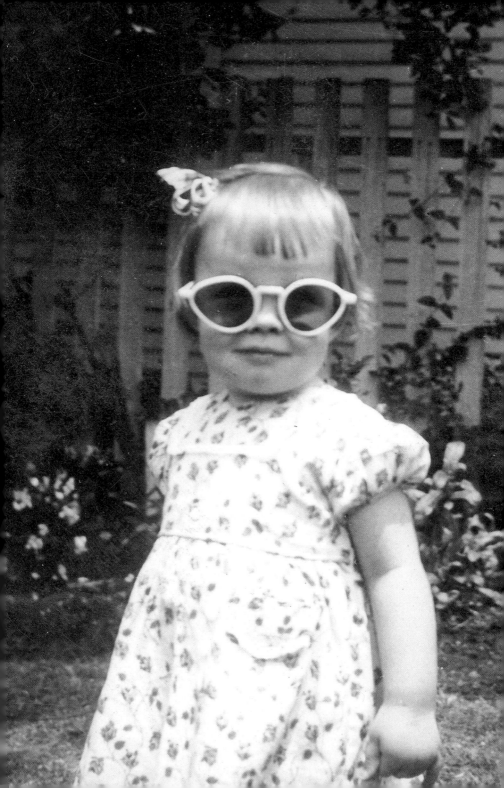

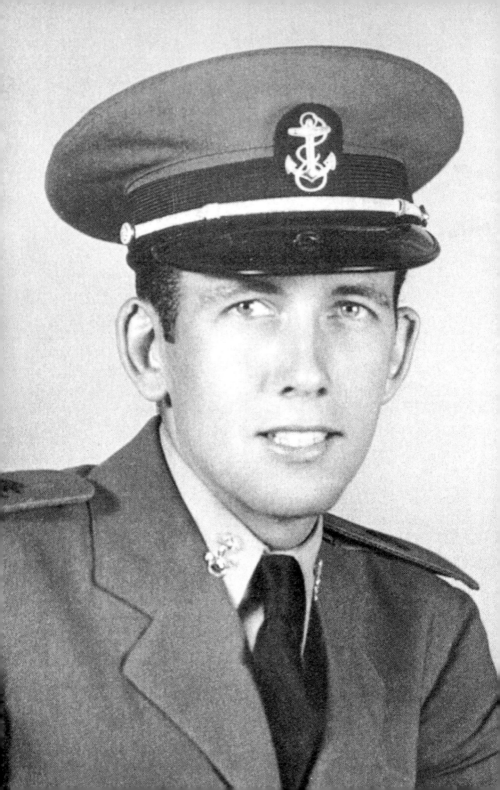

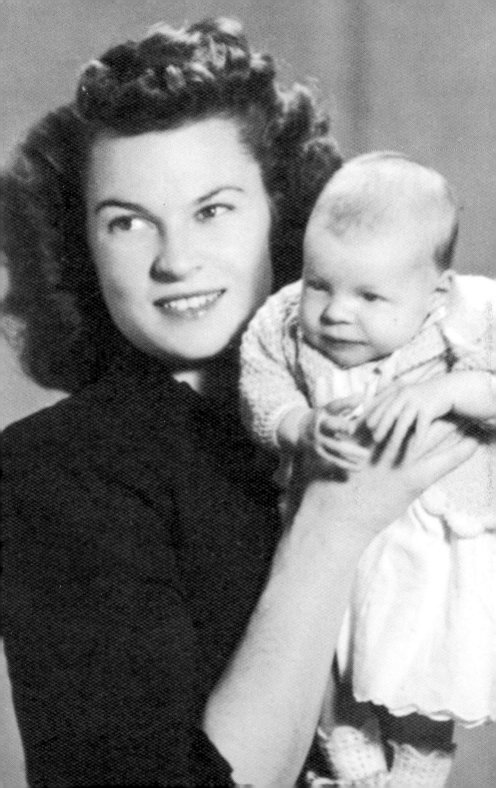

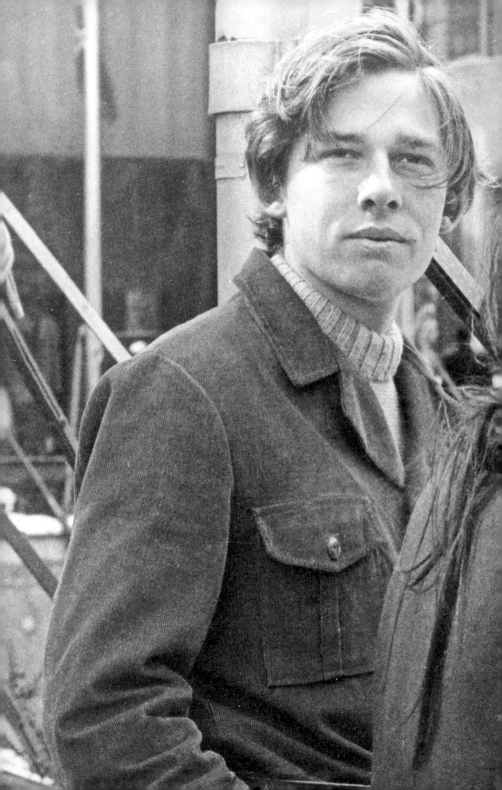

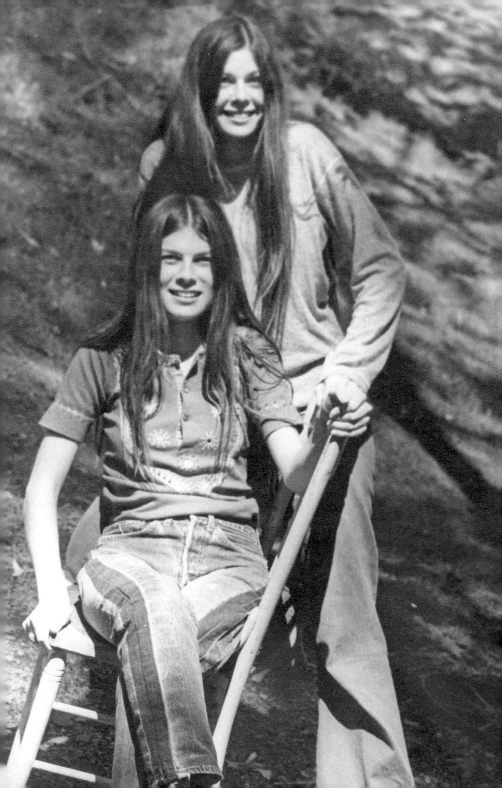

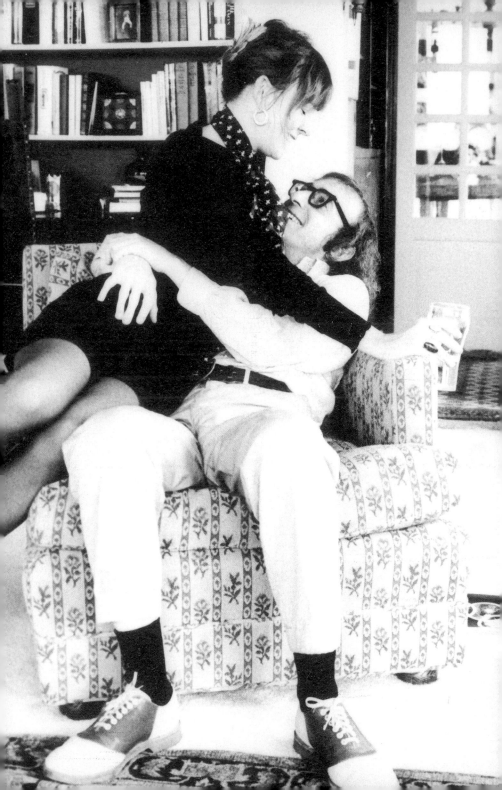

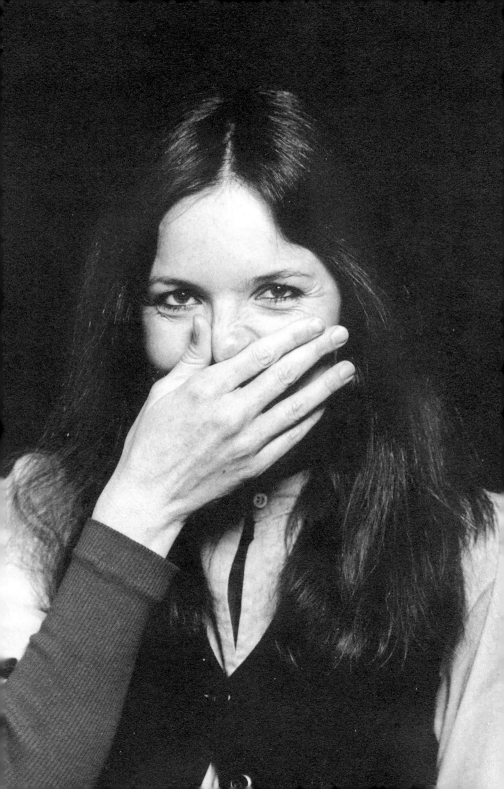

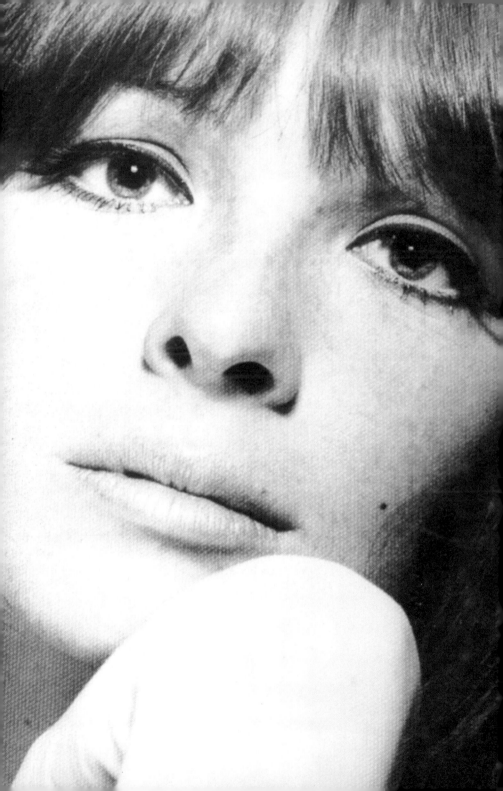

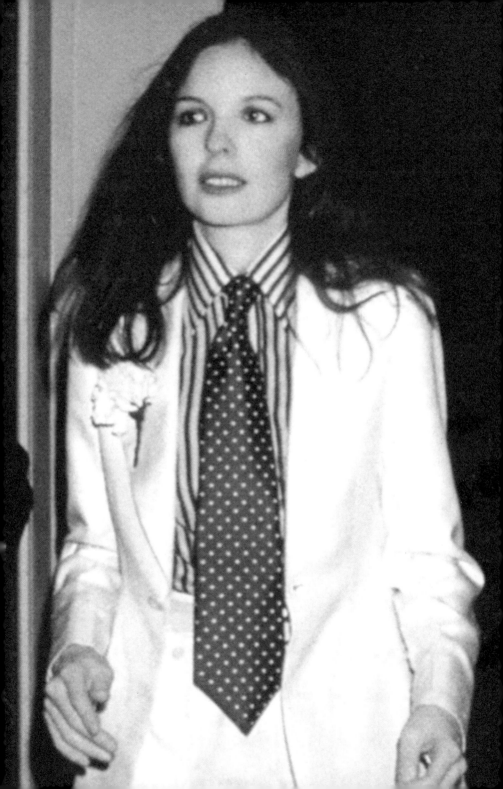

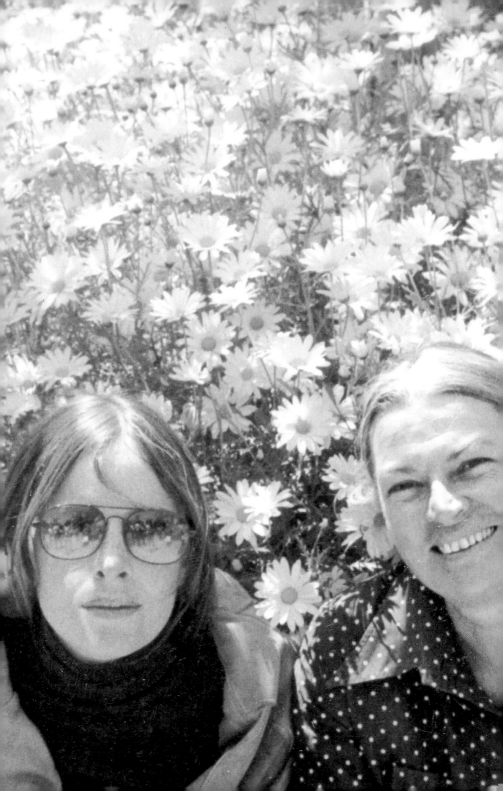

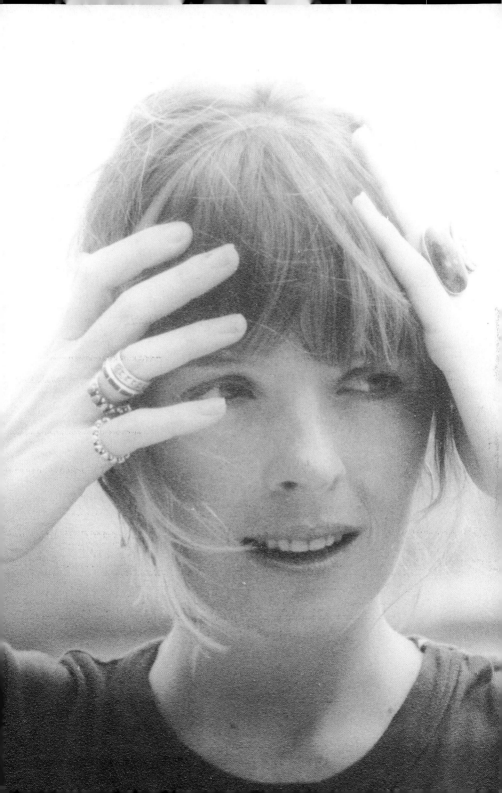

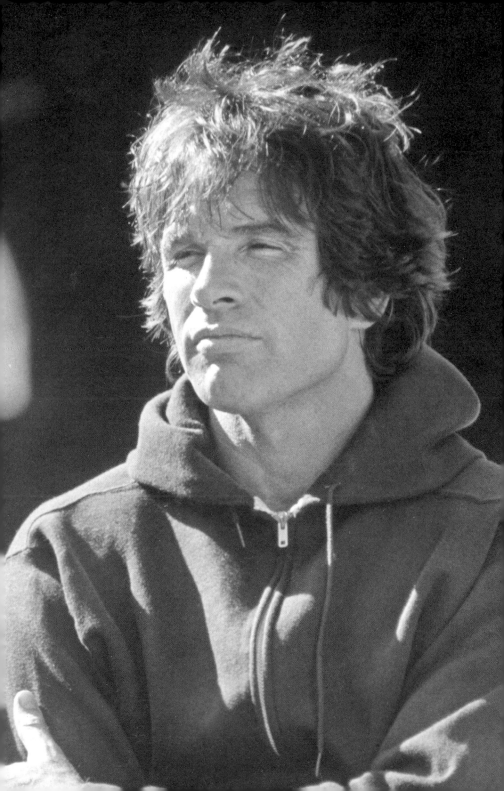

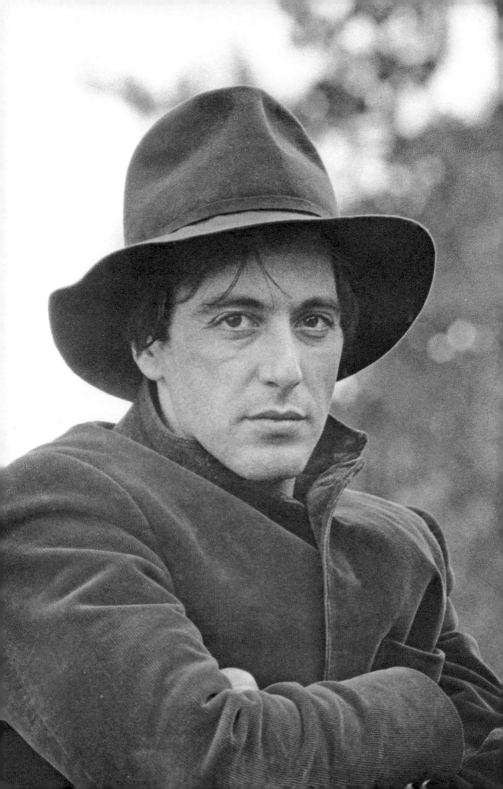

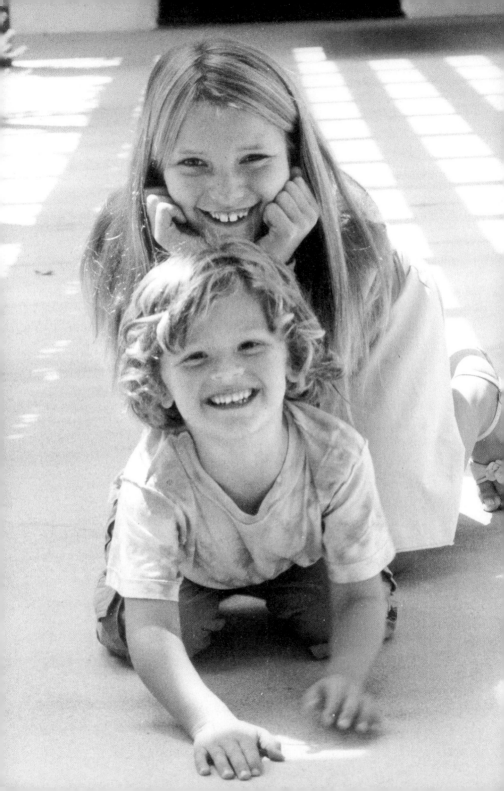

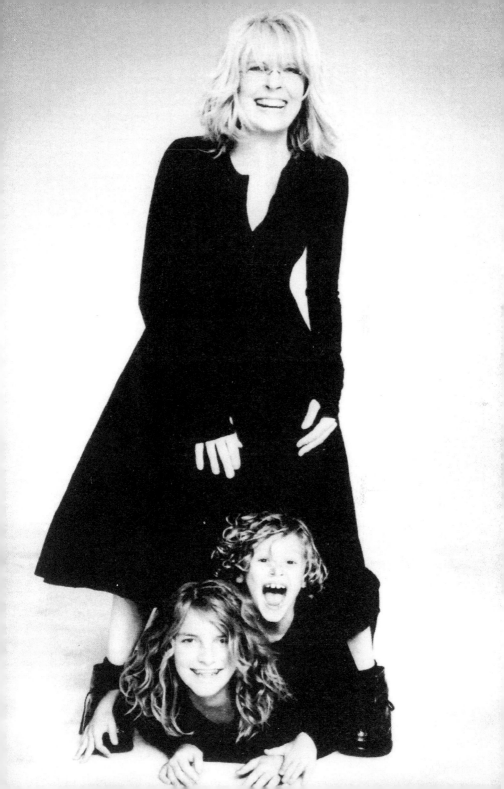

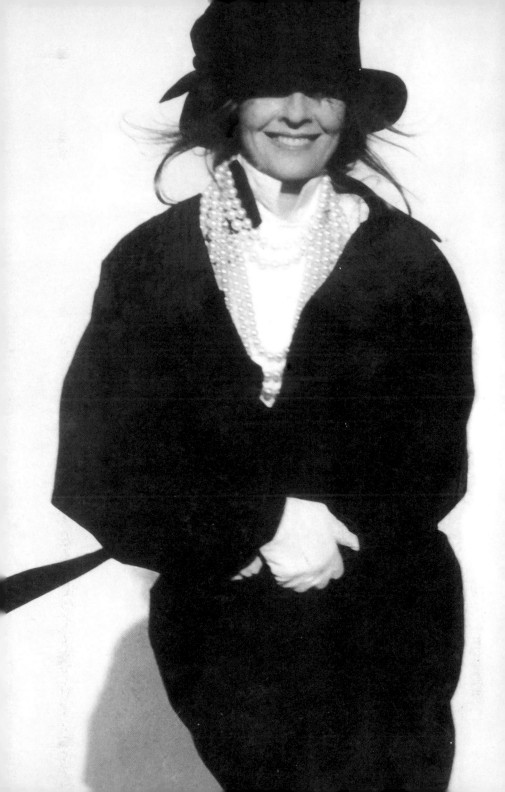

From someone who admired you at a distance last night. Who would like to get to know you better.
Warren

He lived in a four-hundred-square-foot penthouse on top of the Beverly Wilshire Hotel stacked to the ceiling with books and scripts, tons of scripts. It was an unassuming bachelor pad sitting on some of the best real estate in Beverly Hills. He owned an art deco house on ten acres at the top of Mulholland Drive, which he was going to restore into the perfect home. Warren and the notion of home were not a match made in heaven. Always curious, he solicited my design ideas by driving me up into Coldwater Canyon. As he pointed out Jack Nicholson's gate on the right and the panoramic view of L.A. on the left, I heard ringing from what appeared to be a large box. Warren put it to his ear and started talking. It was a car phone, maybe the first.

I listened to him broker a deal with Charlie Bluhdorn, the head of Paramount Pictures, as the smell of stale vitamins from his glove compartment distracted me from the fact that waiting would be my future with "The Pro." It was impossible to drag him away from a phone, a restaurant, a meeting, a club, you name it. Jack Nicholson's solution was to make arrangements to meet Warren at noon, knowing he would arrive at two. I didn't know how to schedule my life like that. Instead, I paced back and forth on the terrace of the Beverly Wilshire or sat waiting on the rented white furniture in his unfinished masterpiece, wondering what happened to the series of failed architects whose drawings and plans were stacked everywhere. How did I ever get to the top of the hill with Warren Beatty anyway? Did he love me, or was I destined to be one of many women who would be driven to the top only to be dropped off at the bottom?

Warren was always working on something but tormented by the prospect of "going to work." He forced himself to make *Heaven Can Wait,* his co-directorial debut with Buck Henry. It was a phenomenal success and landed him on the cover of *Time* magazine, but it didn't change his approach. He still had hundreds of projects in varying states of preparation with people like Buck, Robert Towne, and Elaine May. There was the Howard Hughes script, the remake of *An Affair to Remember,* and the one he kept mentioning about a couple of Communists. Warren's problem was commitment. Dustin Hoffman once said, "If Warren had stayed a virgin, he'd be known as the best director in the world."

On his arm, I was ushered into the homes of people like Katharine Graham, Jackie Kennedy, Barry Diller, Diane von Furstenberg, Jack Nicholson, Anjelica Huston, Sue Mengers, Diana Vreeland, Gay and Nan Talese. I held my own for a while but never quite passed the savvy/smarts/endurance test. In the midst of such remarkable people, I would long to go back to the open arms of my family. I had a few healthy instincts, but I didn't have the fortitude to prolong my moment in the sun. I preferred retreating.

8

SOMETHING BIG
FOR A SMALL FAMILY

Black and White

I was having my portrait taken by Irving Penn for the cover of *Vogue* magazine when an assistant rushed in to announce he'd heard I'd been nominated for an Academy Award. I didn't know how to respond. I'd always thought a nomination would play out like winning Mrs. Highland Park did for Mom. A curtain would open to an audience of thousands applauding, while a crown was placed on my head as I stood surrounded by a new wardrobe, a Cadillac Seville, and keys to a home in Encino. Instead, I was sitting in front of a white backdrop, worrying about the stylist's offhanded remark about my shoulders being too small to wear a strapless gown. She pulled no punches. Mr. Penn's brilliance, as well as his aristocratic manner, didn't fill me with confidence either. When the makeup artist told me the right side of my face was probably better than the left, I forgot all about the fact that my biggest teenage dreams had come true—I was a movie star and Warren Beatty was my boyfriend.

Being familiar enough with Irving Penn's genius, I knew a black-and-white cover would be amazing. How I got the gumption to try to sell *Vogue* the idea is still hard to believe. I had no clout. But I drove a hard bargain. It was black and white or nothing. *Vogue* passed. And that was it. Needless to say, opportunities with *Vogue* did not come up again. I repeated the same demand when I posed for the cover of *Newsweek* in 1980 before the opening of *Reds*. I actually asked Richard Avedon if he would take a few black-and-white photographs along with the color. He did. When the contact sheets arrived, sure enough, the black-and-white close-ups were better. I begged *Newsweek* to use them. I even called Avedon to see if I could enlist his help in my struggle to win. *Newsweek* went with the color. In 2009, thirty years later, I finally landed a black-and-white cover for *More* magazine. Ruven Afanador was the photographer.

February 23, 1978

I heard over radio KRAC that Diane has been nominated for Best Actress for Annie Hall. *So many loose nerve endings. I couldn't settle down. What a state to be in, all alone. This news should have been shared, like when I heard Robin passed the state exam, or like when Randy got pub-*

lished in a major magazine, or like when I got a photo job, or like when Jack succeeded, or Dorrie found a job on her own, like that. But I was alone, so what could I do? I called Jack. Then I called Diane. She wasn't home. When she finally called me later, she couldn't talk long, because Irving Penn was photographing her for a Vogue cover coming up soon.

Sunday night we are scheduled to go out to eat with Diane and Warren Beatty. How will I know what to say to Warren Beatty, how to act, what to wear? Think of it. His sister is nominated. His girlfriend is nominated. What will he do? Where will his loyalties lie? We will be limousined to the music center on Oscar Night. Dorrie will go with Diane, sitting separately. The rest of us will be together in one row, and we'll all go to the party afterwards. I could hardly sleep.

High Heels with Socks

When I told Grammy Hall I'd been nominated for an Academy Award, she shook her head. "That Woody Allen is too funny-looking to pull some of that crap he pulls off, but you can't hurt a Jew, can you? How's Dorothy doing anyway? She looks tired, and your Dad's getting gray fast worrying about Randy. I still don't know what his poetry means anyhow. There's no rhyme to it. Say, are you still seeing that Beatty? Yeah, I'd stick to the guy with money. He's a pretty still fellow, that Beatty though. He's awfully artificial-looking, and he's a womanizer too, ain't he?"

Without a stylist (I didn't know what a stylist was) I drove to Rodeo Drive and hit the stores in Beverly Hills. I knew I couldn't get away with a hat, so I decided to give the layered look all my attention. At Ralph Lauren I bought a vest and two full skirts made of linen. I picked up a pair of fancy slacks to wear underneath at Armani, where I also found a linen jacket, a crisp white shirt, a black string tie, and, of course, a scarf to punch it all up. I bought a belt from Georgio's. And I borrowed a pair of Robin's socks to wear with the high heels I purchased from Saks. It was *Annie Hall* all the way.

That night I dreamed my caps became translucent. Buckets of water leaked in through a hole where the gums hit the porcelain. In order to be ready for the awards ceremony, I had to stand on my head to drain the liquid for twenty-four hours and missed the show.

D-Day

Dorrie and I got out of the limo to bandstand platforms full of screaming people. Kirk Douglas spoke into Army Archerd's microphone as he waved to the crowd. The frenzy of outstretched arms couldn't have cared less about Kirk Douglas. They were shouting for the attention of a twenty-four-year-old stunner named John Travolta, approaching his first big moment on the red carpet. That's what I noticed. Nothing lasts.

The three-hour ceremony was endless anxiety. Midway through, I snuck to the lobby, where I caught Richard Burton smoking a cigarette. He looked up and said something about doubting he would ever win one of "these damn things." I nodded. What else could I do? I was standing next to a legend. He was right. He didn't win. Richard Dreyfuss did. The image of Dreyfuss slapping his hands and pumping his fists was hard to top, but the encounter with Richard Burton's face up close and personal had more staying power. I guess losing is a more human experience.

At the time it didn't dawn on me how inappropriate I looked in my "la de da" layered getup, set against the backdrop of gorgeous women in spectacular gowns. Out of the corner of my eye, I spotted Jane Fonda. Oh, my God. Who was I kidding? I wasn't better than Jane Fonda or Anne Bancroft or Shirley MacLaine or Marsha Mason. They were fabulous.

Dorrie sat next to me and it helped, but I didn't know where I was, or who I was, or how I got there, or what to say. When I heard the *D* sound in a first name that became *Diane*, I still wasn't sure, but I got up anyway and more or less rushed to the podium. I knew winning had nothing to do with being the "best" actress. I knew I didn't deserve it. And I knew I'd won an Academy Award for playing an affable version of myself. I got it. But the fact that *Annie Hall,* a comedy, won best picture thrilled me. For some unfathomable reason, comedy is invariably relegated to the position of second cousin to drama. Why? Humor helps us get through life with a modicum of grace. It offers one of the few benign ways of coping with the absurdity of it all. Looking back, I'm so happy and so grateful and so proud to be in a Great American Comedy.

My first fabulous woman, the most fabulous woman of all, had been "Miss Hepburn at Home" on the cover of *Life* magazine in 1953. As pictured, Audrey was the personification of beauty, with a splash of innocence and awe mixed in. She took my breath away. The impact of such a casual, unassuming, yet stunning photograph must have been the inspiration for my obsession with black-and-white covers. You can imagine my shock when Audrey Hepburn rushed up to me after I won the Academy Award and told me the future was mine. "Really, oh, I don't know. Wow. I don't know about that, I mean the future and all, but you're . . . you . . . you're my idol, I'm just . . . what can I say? I'm so honored to meet you." I stumbled and bumbled. What could I do? This was not "Miss Hepburn at Home." This woman was old.

Everything else about the Academy Awards has all but disappeared. I've forgotten the ball, the congratulations, the fun, even who was there. What remains is Richard Burton and Audrey Hepburn. Nothing could have prepared me for the loneliness on his face or the elegance with which Miss Hepburn handed over the mantle of "movie star." It was almost as if in a camera's flash, Richard Burton had become a broken man, and Audrey Hepburn, my one true without equal, beyond compare, second to none, was no longer a perfect still life.

Audrey Hepburn was sixty-three when she died of cancer. She was forty-eight when I met her, not exactly what you'd call old. Backstage, I pretended to listen to her words, but in truth I couldn't get my mind off age and what it does to a person. Maybe it was said best by Cher: "There is only value to having the look you have when you are young and no value to the look you have when you are older." Instead of taking the time to have a conversation with Audrey Hepburn, I chose to hightail my way out of her company as fast as I could. It is another regret in a growing list of regrets.

Woody woke up the morning after and opened *The New York Times*. On the front page he read that *Annie Hall* won best picture and went back to work on his next script, *Interiors,* a drama. Woody stood by his principles. To him there was no "best" in an art form—that included no best director, no best picture, and definitely no best actress. Art was not a Knicks basketball game.

Even Grammy Hall was interviewed by the local Highland Park newspaper. She had her picture taken with a photograph of Woody in her right hand and one of me in the left. "People say I'm in the clouds, I ain't in no clouds. I'll tell you one thing about the Academy Awards. It's something big for a small family. That Woody Allen must be awfully broadminded to think of all that crap he thinks of."

2009

Before I opened my computer in the parking lot today, I relived one of my favorite memories. It's the one with Woody and me sitting on the steps of the Metropolitan Museum after it's closed. We're watching people parade out of the museum in summer shorts and sandals. The trees to the south are planted in parallel lines. The water in the fountain shoots up with a mist that almost reaches the steps we sit on.

We look at silver-haired ladies in red-and-white-print dresses. We separate the mice from the men, the tourists from the New Yorkers, the Upper East Siders from the West Siders. The hot-pretzel vendor sells us a wad of dough in knots with clumps of salt stuck on top. We make our usual remarks about the crazies and wonder what it would be like to live in a penthouse apartment on Fifth Avenue overlooking the Met. We laugh and say the same things we always say. We hold hands and keep sitting, just sitting, as the sun begins to set. It's a perfect afternoon. There were many perfect afternoons with Woody.

Woody never chose to join me in the sad-sack nostalgia of temporal concerns. He didn't regret the past or try to bring back perfect afternoons that most likely weren't perfect except in memory. He's never spoken of his Academy Awards with an ounce of pride. He doesn't speak of them at all. Even funny is preferred without sentiment. He loves to dish it out. And the deal is, nobody does it better than Woody. He's mastered the put-down. I just wish he would do it more often, like he did at my Lincoln Center honor a few years back.

Lincoln Center Tribute

"I got a call asking if I would say some nice things about Diane. I said, Yes, I can think of some nice things. Keaton for one thing is punctual. She, she, she'll always show up on time, and she's thrifty; she knows the value of a dollar. She, um . . . what else can I say about her . . . She has wonderful handwriting. She's . . . I'm reaching. Uh . . . She's, uh, beautiful. She was always beautiful. She's remained beautiful over the years. She's not beautiful in the conventional sense of the word *beauty*. By the conventional sense I mean 'pleasing to the eye.' She has great conviction in her own taste. She always dresses with the black clothes and the hat and the sensible shoes. She looks to me like the woman who comes to take Blanche DuBois to the institution. It's grammatically incorrect to say someone is 'the most unique' or 'so unique,' but, you know, Diane is the most unique person that I've ever known. That could be interpreted as weirdness but she's, you know, she's truly one of a kind . . . I think."

I miss Woody. He would cringe if he knew how much I care about him. I'm smart enough not to broach the subject. I know he's borderline repulsed by the grotesque nature of my affection. What am I supposed to do? I still love him. I'll always be his Lamphead, Monster, Cosmo Piece, his simple-is-as-simple-does housemeat, and Major Oaf. How do I tell "Uncle Woodums" about my lurve, I mean loave, I mean loof? How can I tell him to please "take care of all your fingers and toes and think sweet thoughts, write if you get a chance, and hang by your thumbs"?

Annie Hall changed my life. When the movie proved to have the kind of legs I'd fantasized but couldn't envision . . . I made a U-turn and withdrew. As much as I appreciated the accolades, I wasn't prepared for the discomfort—or, rather, the guilt—that came with it. I tried going back home. I drove down to my parents' new house on Cove Street at the beach in Corona del Mar. I hung out with Mom. We took pictures of suburbia with our new Nikon F's. Dorrie and I went to swap meets. Randy was writing, and Robin was employed as a visiting nurse caring for the elderly. Warren was getting more serious about directing the love story of John Reed and Louise Bryant set against the Russian Revolution.

I went back to New York and hung out with my friends Kathryn Grody and Carol Kane. What did I think I would get by refusing all the attention I had wanted for so long? This new life was scary. Instead of taking it head-on, I tried to deny fame for as long as I could—maybe too long.

Woody's first drama fit right into my program of avoidance. *Interiors* was, let's just say, not commercial. Miscast as a brilliant writer in the vein of Renata Adler, I smoked cigarettes and knotted my brow in an effort to seem intelligent. The words Woody wrote didn't fit on the lips of my experience. The only things that distracted me from my discomfort in the role were legendary Geraldine Page and Sandy Meisner's favorite actress, Maureen Stapleton.

Every morning Geraldine Page trudged to the set in rags, lugging two shopping bags full of mending. She'd bend over, pull out her husband Rip Torn's old clothes, and patch his pants while she was in the makeup chair. I couldn't wrap my mind around the fact that one of the greatest actresses in the world was a bag lady. If anything, her homeless appearance added to her charisma. When Woody gave her direction, she smiled, nodded her head politely, then completely disregarded everything he said. Before one of her extremely emotional close-ups, I stood next to the camera, about to feed her my lines, when she point-blank asked me to leave. As I watched from a distance, I understood. My presence would have stolen her freedom. Maybe all that Neighborhood Playhouse sharing with your fellow actors, all that living truthfully together in the given imaginary moment, wasn't for everyone. Geraldine Page was an acting genius. Rules don't apply to genius.

Maureen Stapleton, on the other hand, had the appearance of a more predictable approach. She wanted the other actors to be there for her close-ups. With her big round Irish face, Maureen seemed to be suspended in a permanent state of surprise, or frenzy. How did she do it so effortlessly? No one knew. At the end of shooting one day, I waited for her in the teamster van. She was a big woman. Her body didn't have much give, but she managed to lift it into the seat next to me and said, "Someday you'll be old too, Diane."

The solitary year of shooting *Reds* in England was an emotional two steps back and no steps forward. I wasn't prepared for playing Louise Bryant, someone far less romantic than I'd imagined. She became my cross to bear. I didn't like her. There was nothing charming about her will to be recognized as an artist in her own right. Her pursuit of the magnetic revolutionary John Reed was suspect and, frankly, laced with envy. I hated her. It was a problem. Rather than face the challenge, I did what I usually do under pressure: I backpedaled.

On the set, Barry, the hairdresser, would joke about farts while rolling my hair in curlers, as thirtyish Paul slapped on the makeup. Occasionally Jeremy Pikser, one of the writers, would join me for lunch and talk about iconic characters he couldn't stand, like Scarlett O'Hara, who was nothing more than a selfish brat. I don't know, I probably got the message wrong, but it seemed like he was trying to tell me something.

Everyone knew I didn't take well to Warren's direction. It was impossible to work with a perfectionist who shot forty takes per setup. Sometimes it felt like I was being stun-gunned. Even now I can't say my performance is my own. It was more like a reaction to Warren—that's what it was: a response to the effect of Warren Beatty.

It took the tragic reunion of John Reed and Louise Bryant at the train station for me to find a sense of pride in playing such a provocative character. Warren waited through something like sixty-five excruciating close-ups before I finally broke through my self-imposed wall of defiance and let go of my judgment call on a woman I needed to love in order to play. Shooting the scene was an experience I couldn't have foreseen. Because of Warren's tenacity, suddenly, against all odds, love came rushing through when Louise Bryant saw John Reed's face approaching hers at last. *Reds* was an epic with themes enriched by human ideals. John Reed sacrificed his life for his beliefs. But for me, it was imperfect love that was at the heart of Warren's movie.

PART THREE

9

ARTISTIC

Focus

It was the eighties. I was nominated for an Academy Award for *Reds* but lost to Katharine Hepburn in *On Golden Pond*. My next movie, *Shoot the Moon,* was released to mixed critical success. *The Little Drummer Girl* tanked big-time. *Mrs. Soffel* with Mel Gibson also bombed. Beth Henley's *Crimes of the Heart,* with Jessica Lange and Sissy Spacek, was sweet but did little business. Somehow, Martin Scorsese and Robert De Niro agreed to have a meet/greet for their upcoming film *Cape Fear.* They went with Jessica Lange. Other projects, including *Almost Human, Reform School, Klepto, Whatever Happened to Harry,* and *Book of Love,* never saw the light of day.

It's not that I didn't work. I worked in Canada, Los Angeles, Finland, Spain, Russia, Great Britain, Greece, Napa,

Israel, Germany, and Southport, North Carolina. It's just that for the most part my contribution to the art of filmmaking wasn't particularly inspired. When I wasn't on the road I continued to live in New York. Warren, having won his Oscar for best director, was here and there, until there won out. Woody met Mia Farrow and began a new alliance. Without a great man writing and directing for me, I was a mediocre movie star at best. I didn't have a publicist. I chose not to brand out with an Annie Hall line of clothes. I didn't have a manager, nor did I want one anymore.

When I wasn't acting, I pursued a variety of visual hobbies under the umbrella of "art." My friend Daniel Wolf even agreed to give me a show of paintings based on religious pamphlets I'd collected at swap meets. I commissioned a Kansas City sign painter named Robert Huggins to put my ideas on several billboard-size canvases. When *Religious Commissions* proved to be inexplicably bizarre, I took photographs à la Sandy Skoglund, most famous for *Radioactive Cats,* which features green-painted clay cats running amok in a gray kitchen. In honor of Sandy, I assembled a tableau setting in my living room that resembled the view from an alpine ski lodge, complete with fake rocks bought at a prop shop and genuine-looking crows flying overhead. Nine willing ballerinas in pink tutus and masks agreed to stand in front of my homemade diorama and have their photograph taken. It became glaringly apparent I was no Sandy Skoglund, so I took portraits of friends like Carol Kane sitting inside boxes with polka dots framing their faces under patterned light casting shadows. I also wrote lyrics to songs that were never recorded. "She sits in a Chinese restaurant.

She's crappy. She's a creep; she looks at him. She's lost too much sleep. And a one, and a two, a one two three. Two different worlds . . . We live in two different worlds . . . Our hearts . . ." Et cetera. I started photographing people on the streets, à la Diane Arbus. As if that wasn't enough, I began cutting and pasting four-by-six-foot collages. One, called *Face Lift Off,* featured Bette Davis's head being hoisted up into God knows where. Don't ask.

Warren, now a friend, would remind me I was a movie star. Focus on that. I didn't listen. Cindy Sherman had arrived on the scene and, with her, the decade of appropriation. I wanted to be part of it. I kept telling myself I was an artist. The awful truth was, no matter how hard I tried, I was an actress who hadn't been in a comedy since *Manhattan* in 1979.

On the Road

I took some of Warren's advice and went looking for a movie to produce. After reading *Somebody's Darling,* the story of one of the few bankable female directors in Hollywood and her best friend, I took the train to Washington, D.C., and met my own soon-to-be-friend Larry McMurtry at his store Booked Up. Larry, with his feet on the desk, listened to my pitch. Not skipping a beat, he said he'd give me the option *and* he'd write the script too. Six months later it was finished. That's the kind of guy Larry is. My agent secured a meeting with Sherry Lansing, the head of Paramount, who did not mince words when she told me the project was not

commercial. That was it for *Somebody's Darling,* but not for
my friendship with Larry.

Every other month or so, I would hop on the Amtrak to
D.C., where Larry and I would hit the streets in his Cadillac.
As usual, I had a creative task that consumed me. One time
it revolved around a series of photographs on taxidermied
animals. Leave it to Larry to know some people who owned
a pair of stuffed sheep joined at the hip. Traveling became a
metaphor for our friendship.

On one of our road trips through Texas, I told Larry
about my dream of living in Miami Beach, where it was forever humid and hot. Sometimes, I told him, I thought about
moving to Atlantic City or Baja California. Then again,
what I really wanted to do was pack it in and move to Pasadena near the arroyo, right by Greene and Greene's Gamble
House. Larry listened with a Dr Pepper in one hand, the
steering wheel in the other. When we found ourselves on the
outskirts of Ponder, Texas, a big sign told us that *Bonnie and
Clyde* had been shot within the city limits. Warren Beatty—
my high school crush; my Splendor in the Grass. It was impossible to wrap my mind around the fact that we met,
became intimate, and spent a year making *Reds.* Drifting
back to 1967, I remembered Mom's home movie of *Bonnie
and Clyde,* starring Randy as C. W. Moss, Robin as Bonnie,
Dorrie as Blanche, and me, Diane, as Clyde Barrow. I had
outright refused to be Bonnie. Hell, no. I didn't want to be
Bonnie. I was going to be Warren Beatty. Who in their right
mind wouldn't? And that became our central problem. I
wanted to be Warren Beatty, not love him.

The facts of my life felt more surreal than any dream. As

we passed through Ponder, I rolled down the window. Out of the dust that enveloped our silence, Larry's words started coming and going. "It's so plain in Nebraska, I can't tell you, it's just totally plain. Last week I crossed the Missouri on a tiny toll bridge and the little old woman toll keeper was so lonely, she made me stop and eat a doughnut with her. 'It's punk here in the wintertime,' she said. 'I sit here all day just grinding my teeth.'" Then he'd be quiet for a while and begin again. Larry was a born storyteller. I think about those times, the lull of the engine, the endless horizon, and Larry's words dangling. It turned out we shared something the filming of *Somebody's Darling* could never have given us: a friendship and the road.

Memories

Dear Diane,

My book has a total of three pages. So far my diggings have turned up a bit of pain I can't avoid but funny remembrances too. Many thoughts I kept so private dwell on my anger toward authority figures that never came out as anger. Writing this is not a pleasant pastime; in fact the book is seldom touched, because I'm trying to be accurate & honest.

I'm not writing about the years you kids were growing up. I don't want to be guilty of "the good ole days" trap. All I need to do is sift through the photos of us, and I sink into a nostalgia of the WORST kind. In Memories *it's not like that; I'm writing of things that shaped me. I remember a common thought I had about not doing things my parents did when I grew up. I would make chocolate instead of yellow cake. I would laugh & talk a lot. I would keep romantic love alive. I would be loving rather than impatient with my kids. I thought these CHANGES WOULD take place—*

It's a day to speak of today—so sparkly & beautiful—Jack bought himself a 12 ft. sailboat yesterday. He is happy. We will be sailing later. I have a strong feeling of fun ahead.

Love,

Mom

Mother didn't finish her memoir, *Memories*. Memories. Lost memories. Memories unfinished. A book called *Memories*. It was almost as if God's will had taken over Mother's future. I didn't notice. I was too busy to register the significance of taking on the task of writing a memoir or to be encouraging enough to help. I don't know if I actually read Mother's letter. I have no recollection. I was content to assume Mom was free from the drama of raising us kids and now she had all the time she needed to devote to her artistic pursuits. Of course, I made sure I didn't know what was going on. I had other more important things on my mind.

Sometimes this house is so quiet—I can't figure how it got to be, or why. I walk around as if looking for noise. I speak to the cats, one at a time, or together. The windows draw me to look out; around the yard; check the pool; is the light still on or off? At another time this oversight drove me crazy. Where are all those things and people who brought their sounds to me? I don't mind being alone. I like it most of the time. When it closes in on me a touch too much, I just walk out of the place, get in the car, and go for a drive.

Seeing as a Way of Being

After ten years in New York, things continued to stand out, like the photograph *Woman Seen from the Back* by Onésipe Aguado, at the Met. What does she see facing the wrong direction? I wanted to see it too. The picture was taken in the nineteenth century, yet the distance between her past and my present seemed to collapse. It's hard to believe a woman's back made it clear that seeing rather than being seen could be something so extraordinary, but it did. The power of photography's ability to evoke rather than explain inspired me. Nothing has changed. Books like *Now Is Then, The Waking Dream,* and *Least Wanted* are links to artists who forged a path into their imagination. At least, that's what it seems like to me.

Marvin Heiferman was the director of Castelli Graphics when he gave me a little show of photographs I had taken in hotel lobbies around the United States. "Reservations" included photographs of a broken-down, empty Ambassador Hotel, where Mom had been crowned Mrs. Los Angeles; the Stardust Hotel lobby, where Dad invested and lost every penny when I was twelve years old; the Fontainebleau in Miami Beach; the Pierre in New York; and the Biltmore in Palm Springs.

Thanks for Nothing

A few years later, Marvin and I decided to collaborate on a book of publicity shots from old movies. It took us to basements and warehouses throughout Los Angeles, where we hunted down large-format photographs of movie stars posed in scenes from *South Pacific, Lassie,* and *Bigger Than Life,* with James Mason, to name a few. Plowing through thousands of discarded four-by-five-inch color transparencies, I couldn't help but wonder what had happened to Joan Crawford, James Mason, Annette Funicello, and even Elvis. Inanimate and waxy, they looked like the taxidermied animals from the series of photographs I had taken with Larry.

I knew I was on to something major with the stuffed-animal motif. It made me think of that Roy Rogers quote, "I told Dale, 'When I go, just skin me and put me on top of Trigger.'" Which in turn gave me the idea of a title, *Still Life.* Get it? My favorite example was the photograph of Gregory Peck from *The Man in the Gray Flannel Suit.* I even wrote him into my introduction.

It's hard to love someone you've never known, but it's easy to long for someone you've seen idealized to the point where you think you're in love. When you grow up, you're supposed to be able to distinguish between fantasy and real affection. For instance, I know Gregory Peck isn't going to enter my life and become an intimate part of it. Most people know that, and by the time they reach adulthood, they don't want Gregory Peck anymore. But if Gregory Peck touched them once—he touched me once—he remains a very vital part of their makeup. The ideal image of him takes on many dimensions. He becomes a representation of the frequently frustrated longings of adolescence, all those things you wanted to believe life was going to place at your feet.

After *Still Life* was published I received a letter from Gregory Peck. He wasn't pleased. He thought the book was stupid. On top of that he didn't appreciate being compared to a stuffed animal. It was such a lame, kitschy idea, he hoped I wasn't the mastermind behind it. He ended by saying my heartfelt introduction was total crap.

It never entered my mind that Gregory Peck might feel bad about looking almost real in front of a fake backdrop. I was busy patting myself on the back for a book Gregory Peck dismissed as camp, and how, miracle of miracles, it captured the essence of taxidermy and how it was going to put me on the map—which one I'm not sure.

Gregory Peck is on my long list of regrets I hope to be forgiven for. I'm sorry I carelessly held him accountable for some publicist's brainstorm. I'm sorry I picked an iconic photograph that shed light on his stiff upper lip and abiding lack of affect, which hounded him throughout his career, like my own eccentricity hounds me.

In the Meantime

I talked to a woman at Hunter's Bookstore who had just spent 3 days cleaning out her deceased aunt's huge Victorian house. The aunt, a spinster, had died at age 86. She saved everything ever given, sent, or found. When asked why, she said that it gave her pleasure. She wouldn't care what happened to it after she died. Her niece bought a box of heavy-duty trash bags and without sympathy pitched all of it into the dump. It was as if I was hearing this for a specific reason. All the writing I do, and all the words on paper I put away, and all the little inspirational messages I cut and save that I feel were written and directed to me and me alone, don't matter. After I'm gone, I won't care whether the family reads any of it or tosses all of it in the dump. There are some words I would want them to read though: the ones detailing my thoughts and feelings about each of them; how much I loved them, what it was about them that was so special to me; those five people who will be doing the pitching.

Imagining Heaven, the Ultimate Coming Attraction, 1987

It took a year and a half to make my documentary, *Heaven*. The reception was unanimous. I suppose the most painful rejection came from Vincent Canby of *The New York Times*. "*Heaven,* a film by Diane Keaton, is the cinema equivalent of a book that's discounted to $19.95 before Christmas with the warning that it will be $50 after. If you respond to that kind of come-on, you may respond to *Heaven*. One's torn between wanting to kick the film and wanting to protect it from wasting all this money."

Heaven was a promise I'd longed for as a little girl. I knew I was afraid to die, but if I had to, I wanted to go to heaven. The epiphany came thirty years later, when I visited the Mormon Tabernacle visitors' center in Salt Lake City with my friend Kristi Zea. Entering the dome-shaped hall, we saw what I can only describe as a coming attraction, featuring smiling people in white robes floating in the sky. Even Kristi agreed it was a strange juxtaposition of images that could inspire only a surrealist. I may not have been a surrealist, but I was inspired. I called my producing partner Joe Kelly. I had an idea.

We got permission to see 16-millimeter copies of MGM heaven-themed features as well as obscure evangelical Super 8 short films. The more I saw, the more my appetite grew, culminating with several visits to the film historian William Everson's apartment in New York, where he screened Dreyer's *The Passion of Joan of Arc,* Cocteau's *Beauty and the Beast,* Fritz Lang's *Liliom* and both *Dr. Mabuse*s—and more. Not only did we gather astonishing footage, we also assembled people who gave heaven the beauty of their imaginations. There was Alfred Robles, Grace Johansen, Don King, and the Reverend Robert Hymers, author of *UFOs and Bible Prophecy* (reprinted as *Encounters of the Fourth Kind*), to name a few.

When Joe and I began shooting interviews, I asked stirring questions like, "Is there sex in heaven?" "Is there love in heaven?" "Are you afraid to die?" Mom and Dad and Grammy Hall were among my first interviews. Dad was convinced. "If there is something after death, and I've led a good life, I can't conceive why Dorothy and I wouldn't be together." Mom nodded her head and said, "It's a subject I don't like to think or give credence to." "Yeah," Dad said, "it's something you don't think about. I have partners that do, but I don't." Grammy Hall summed it up best: "There ain't such a thing as heaven. Have you ever seen anybody who passed away that you loved and wanted to see? No! Nobody ever come back and said, 'Well, here I am and I am so glad to see you.' Anybody tells you they've died and gone to heaven is a dirty liar."

After Paul Barnes, the editor, helped put the movie together, we began the preview process. Apparently the audience best suited to see a movie like *Heaven* came from two groups: women and "experiential" types. It turned out experientials were your "oddballs," your "weirdos," and your "downtown set." This was concerning. Were there enough experiential women from downtown to make our movie a moderate success? We certainly had our fair share appearing in the movie, like the woman who said, "I've seen Jesus in the spirit. He entered my bedroom. He came from the top of the window like you roll the scroll, and he was nothing but a spirit. His chest was made out of sky, and his shoulders were made out of cloud. And he moved just like the waves in the water. All at once I heard a universal harp like . . . ooohhh . . . like a wind blowing oooohhh . . . like the wind when it blows like ooooohhhhh. That's when he flipped over in my room. Then he floated through my bedroom and I said, 'In the bathroom,' so then he went right into the bathroom and then I said, 'In the living room.' He went right into the living room and sat on the ottoman. I said, 'In the kitchen.' But he had to go back through my dining room to get to the kitchen, and he turned and faced me, and when he turned he had on a different outfit with a little hood over his head. And that's the truth.'' It turned out we had more experientials in the movie than in the audience.

No matter how many critics hated *Heaven,* I have to say, I loved every clip and every interview. Spending time trying to make sure I made the smart choice about the right movie to appear in wasn't nearly as entertaining. But *Heaven, Reservations, Still Life,* and even *Religious Commissions* were just that: completely entertaining. I recognize that these projects wouldn't have seen the light of day if it hadn't been for my movie-star status. My forays outside the hub of celebrity felt right, almost like home, not really but sort of.

Found

Heaven brought me something else: Al Pacino one more time. We ran into each other outside an editing bay at the film center where he was working on his 16-millimeter film, *The Local Stigmatic,* while I was finishing up with the hereafter. He was irresistible, as always, and we started palling around, but it was different this time. We were older. He wasn't the Godfather. I wasn't Kay Corleone. We were two people plugging away at a couple of independent films. There was a disheveled aspect to Al that was very appealing, almost familial. He invited me to come to his home one Sunday, then another and another. It was always the same. After the softball game with Al as shortstop, the usual cast of characters—Sully Boyer; Mark, Al's half brother; Adam Strasberg; John Halsey; and Michael Hedges—would drive to his house on the Hudson. The place was filled with activity. Al's three dogs ran around. Stray actors like William Converse Roberts and Christine Estabrook—in pink shorts with matching tank top—would pop in for a few minutes, while Charlie Laughton, Al's mentor, and his wife, Penny, discussed the dying role of the theater. Al would join in with thoughts of doing a workshop of *Salome* or *Macbeth*. These conversations would go on for hours and hours. Al was consumed by two things: baseball and the theater.

He was an artist. He made me think about the difference between being an artist and being artistic. I knew where I stood. I was artistic. For the first time it didn't matter. I just wanted him to love me. I'm pretty sure in Al's mind I was a friend he could talk to. As much as I loved listening, I wanted more, lots of more. Tons. I wanted him to want me as much as I wanted him.

In the middle of this love came *Baby Boom*. The script, about a woman who is forced to adopt a baby, was laugh-out-loud hilarious (or, as Dexter would say, LOL). Charles Shyer and Nancy Meyers, the writing-directing-producing team, were talented and charming. Nancy and my soon-to-be-dear-friend Susie Becker, the costume designer, made me over. It was great to feel attractive and cute and funny again. I became J. C. Wiatt—snappy, sassy, and ready to go. What great good fortune. Or, as J. C. Wiatt would have said, "I'm back. I am back." And it wasn't *Heaven* that did it.

The Future Isn't What It Used to Be

When I arrived at the Glendale Adventist Medical Center, Grammy Hall sat on the side of the hospital bed, ready to go home. Her white hair was pushed back with three rusted bobby pins. Her rayon pants outfit, ablaze with orange, red, and yellow flowers, was offset by the geometric pattern of her blouse, also aflame. "Dorrie's new boyfriend is a Jew. Did you know that, Diane? Also that nurse Holly's fiancé is an Eyetalian. And that new aide is a Lebanon. I think she's a sister to Danny Thomas." "How are you feeling, Gram?" "It seems most of my trouble is in my head. It's that there gland. There's poor circulation in my brain, see. They took X-rays of my head. They seem to think I'm in a bad way. Don't worry, Diane; I lived a long life, too long. I'm not making many future plans, see, 'cause I don't want to live that long. That's too long to live to wait for, what . . . fifteen or twenty dollars?"

I was as close to Mary Hall as she would let me be. And vice versa. She was ninety-four when she died. Back in the fifties, I hadn't cottoned to Grammy Hall. She didn't try to paint a pretty picture of the world. Her Christmas presents were awful: a year's supply of Mission Pack pears delivered to our door every month. Like I cared about pears. It was only when I grew up that I began to respect her.

True, she was unevolved, but she was not a hypocrite.

She was 100 percent honest. She was a practicing skeptic, as well as a practicing Catholic. What a contradiction in terms, especially when you consider she didn't believe in Jesus or heaven. She saw through the pretense and accepted it with a shrug, saying, "It's a long drawn-out proposition, ain't it, Diane. Like I always say, it's the same old sixes or sevens." She died a devout Catholic. Hey, Gram, I'm with you; why not cover all bases, just in case, on the off chance you might be wrong?

Dorothy at Sixty-three

I am a woman of medium height: once five feet eight, now five seven. I keep my records in this leather-bound journal titled 1980. I have no unpaid bills or financial obligations to meet. My present bank account number is 45572 1470. I have four issue (children). Their birth dates are Jan. 5, 1946, March 21, 1948, March 27, 1951, and April 1, 1953. Their names are Diane, Randy, Robin, and Dorrie. I am married to Jack Newton Hall, a citizen of the United States. His eyes are blue. His hair is graying. He is 6 feet tall. We live on a lot, which measures 30 by 40 feet. It is barely big enough to build a house, but we did, and we love it. We have fire and flood insurance. Neither my husband nor I have life insurance. We each drive a car. My car is a silver Jaguar, license number 1FTU749. Jack drives a Toyota mini van, license number JNH on the front with silver letters on a black background. I have signed my last will and testament.

It hereby revokes all other wills or codicils at anytime previously made by me.

I was born in Winfield City, Kansas, in Crowley County. My birth date was October 31, 1921, the year President Harding was sworn into office and Land O'Lakes butter was introduced to the state of New York. My father, Samuel Roy Keaton, a man of medium height, was a sheet metal worker. My mother, Beulah, was a housewife with gray eyes. They had three daughters, Orpha, Martha, and me.

At 63, I have long gray hair. I wash it with Sassoon shampoo. My conditioner is Silkience. I dry it with a Revlon hand held blow dryer. I curl it with Clairol hot rollers. I bathe in HOT water. I brush my teeth with an Oro Flex toothbrush dipped in hydrogen peroxide. My teeth are sound, as is my mind. I try to drink 8 glasses of water each day. I sleep in nighties, under two white blankets with my husband beside me. In the morning I turn on the radio and immediately put on one of four warm robes. There's the one I bought at Macy's N.Y. with Diane for 50 dollars. There's the short one with six snaps down the front that Dorrie got me. There's the pink peachy robe with oriental flower designs all over it. But my favorite is my much worn purple robe from Saks 5th Ave. It really is a part of me. My feelings are wrapped inside it.

My face and neck are fairly wrinkled now. I am giving myself a great deal of personal care these days. I apply cell rejuvenator at night and skin lifter in the morning, followed by wrinkle straightener in between. I was promised a sur-

prise at the end of 15 days. 90 days later, I see no change. I like to keep my face clean and colored up with red cheek rouge, brown eye pencil, and various shades of lipstick. I seldom forget to apply a hearty dose of cologne to my body.

We have radios everywhere, even a new one in my darkroom that tapes from tapes. A blue radio sits in my bathroom window. Jack and I each have a radio on either side of the bed. Our newest radio sits on the white countertop in our white kitchen. Listening to talk radio is a constant. I take Feldene arthritis medication for my hand and jaw. I swallow one capful of Geritol for my vitamin requirement every morning. I wear glasses for reading; one pair in every room I work in.

I've changed in ways beyond my imagination. The lack of physicality has hit with apparent permanency. I sleep more than I did when I was younger. My dreams are evasive when I try to recapture them. I'm content to stay home all day, waiting for Jack and our evening chat with drinks and dinner. I don't need people around. We don't have guests over very much. I've lost my singing voice; even my speaking voice has gone soft and hoarse. I can't play the piano anymore. I don't listen to music. I sit in my darkroom and play solitaire for long periods of time. I spend too much time alone. I get in my car and go out, but I'm always home by 1 o'clock.

After I change into something comfortable I get serious about monitoring the Cove. I watch cars come and go. I see who leaves and where they're going. I study Champ, Jim Beauchamp's wonderful golden retriever. His wife Martha ignores Champ. To me she misses the very essence of that brilliant creature.

There are times I feel as if I'm a true artist. At the moment I'm working on a large sheet of white cardboard I'm transforming into a collage. It's going well, but I tell no one. I have about five completed works framed and ready to go. Two have been accepted in a show at Santa Ana College. I work on the floor of my darkroom, where I spend a lot of time cutting out things I like from the Times. *But I always get my housework done first. It's a habit I can't break. I make the bed, straighten the bathroom, finish the dishes, adjust the pleated blinds at the windows, plan the evening meal, make a list of things to do for that day, get dressed, and then, only then, do I turn to the work in my workroom. Sometimes I can stick with it and sometimes not. It doesn't matter because it's only for me anyway.*

I have no grandchildren. I'm not sure at my advanced age that I want any little copies running around. I don't feel capable of such a responsibility.

My friends are my cats, Perkins and Cyrus. They depend on me for entertainment as well as food and lodging. Being home a lot and having no company but them is an invitation to carry on some interesting conversations. I looked at Perkins in the eye this morning as she was sitting on my bathroom sink, her two lime green eyes locked with mine, and I asked her just what exactly were her goals in life. I was curious. She spends most of the day running from things like footsteps, voices, other cats, people, rain, wind, and radio noise. I wonder how Perkins gets anything worthwhile out of life. Cyrus obeys me when I order him off the

counter, but he doesn't remember to stay off permanently.
He does remember to check out the refrigerator whenever
the door opens. Finally it's clear to me that he remembers
what he wishes to remember. Quite human.

I read the Los Angeles Times *every day,* Newsweek
magazine weekly, and as much fiction as I can squeeze in. I
have an IBM electric typewriter that I use with pleasure. I
keep a daily journal. I like books, cats, nice people, good
food, bourbon and sometimes gin, writing words, being
alone. I LOVE: my husband, my four children, my sisters,
my one day at the bookstore, sunsets, the bay in front of
our house, my Jaguar, Mary Hall (now), and myself (some-
times). I have weekly visits with a psychiatrist, who is try-
ing to help me see myself in a better light. I have two or
three close friends I can talk to openly. Gretchen, Margaret,
and Jo. I go months between visits with them. I don't talk
on the phone much. I don't offer invitations to people, be-
cause I fear rejection. I've been rejected a number of times. I
enjoy working in the darkroom and doing a variety of art
projects, with nothing to show for it, of course. I guess I'm
a fragmented person. I do nothing really well. I have, at the
moment, no motivation.

In Response, Diane at Sixty-three

I'm sixty-three, once five feet seven, now five six. The feelings
and thoughts that overwhelmed Dorothy could and do mirror much of what I feel as well. Advanced age? Oh, yeah.
Good at anything? I can still memorize lines. Do I fear rejec-

tion? I'm an actress. Fragmented? More than most. The difference is—Dorothy at sixty-three was finished raising her four children. At sixty-three, I'm doing what Dorothy did when she was twenty-four.

Yesterday I found Dexter and her new boyfriend of three days, Ben, on video chat. When I confronted her, it was simple: "I'm a video-chat addict, Mom." A video-chat addict? Does that mean she has an addiction to Facebook as well? How else could she have acquired three hundred fifty friends in less than three weeks? There are so many surprising aspects to Dexter, like how brave she was with Dr. Sherwood, her orthodontist, after he finally recognized that the tissue growing over the screw closing the gap from her missing tooth had to be removed, just as she had told me months ago. When we rushed to the oral surgeon, she never uttered a sound while he extracted the tooth. What a sturdy person; how resilient in the face of pain and fear; how unlike me, her anxious mother.

Then there's "Duke's World." Yesterday I picked him up after school. He barely slammed the car door shut before he launched in on how unfair it is that his friend Jasper, age seven, should have an iPhone when he, eight-year-old Duke, does not. Magnanimously, he offered to buy it with his own money. Knowing he doesn't have any money made me admire his chutzpah. When I told him I wanted to think about it, he said, "How long?" "For a while." "When?" "Duke, I'll tell you later." "Tomorrow?" "Duke, enough!" "Tomorrow??" I tuned the radio to 102.7, praying Ryan Seacrest would distract him while I looked at the newly abandoned storefronts in Westwood Village and remembered the call I got from Evelyn, a mother from Dexter's pre-K days who wanted to know if I knew anyone who needed some legal work. Her husband had lost his job. I was trying to think of who I might know, when Ryan Seacrest exceeded my wildest dreams and played Duke's favorite song, "Apple Bottom Jeans." I rejoiced in silence for a full three minutes.

When we pulled up to basketball camp at the YMCA, Duke reminded me he's too big for the booster seat, plus he wanted his usual chocolate mint milk tea warm, not hot, so don't forget the ice cubes, and did I have any Dubble Bubble sugarless gum? As I pulled away, I took one last look at my boy; God, is he beautiful or what? And then, just as I remembered that Carol Kane was going to spend the night, the phone rang. It was my partner Stephanie Heaton. "L'Oreal might want to sponsor the Lifetime screening of *Because I Said So* on Mother's Day." She also reminded me of the speech I hadn't memorized for the Unique Lives speaking engagement coming up. I started worrying.

At sixty-three, I have a daughter who insists she won't swim the 400 IM at the COLA swim meet. She won't. She can't. She does. Duke cries about how his SO MEAN MOM never lets him do anything he wants. At sixty-three there's the morning pill ritual: Dexter's Migravent, for headaches; my miracle Metanx vitamins; our old dog Red's five different capsules for Cushing's disease, among other ailments; Duke's "Biotic," as he calls his vitamins; and our fat dog Emmie's shit-eating pills, which after six months still haven't done the trick. At sixty-three there's still a lot of pleasure, like cleaning out Emmie's earwax and still being allowed to stroke Duke's head in public. The endless struggle to get Dexter to kiss me at least once a week is worth it. The mountain of hugs and kisses makes things way okay. So does the thrill of still being able to give Duke a piggyback ride. The marvel of watching Dexter's intricate nightly beauty regimen is the best way to say goodbye to the day. Good times.

At sixty-three, I can't change into comfortable clothes like Mom and watch the world outside my window. I can't hurry home in retreat from the stress of human contact, as if solitude will bring peace. I know solitude is no one's friend, and retreat is not an option. But I take comfort in the fact that Mother and I will always be bound together by the need to communicate. In spite of the pain of anonymity, Dorothy realized her most valued dream. She wrote. And while she wrote she wasn't criticizing her efforts. She wasn't worried about rejection. She was engaged. She was giving evidence to the experience of being Dorothy Deanne Keaton Hall.

Dad was always telling me to think. Think ahead. Think. Think, Diane. But it was Mom's struggles, her conflicts, and her love that made whatever ability I have to *think* possible. She supported choices that created experiences that expanded my life. As a girl, Mom, like me, had vague grandiose aspirations, but, unlike me, no one helped her expand on them; no one could. It was the poverty of the Depression, not the fabulous fifties. It was Dorothy and Beulah. Then it became Dorothy and Diane.

10

THIS ISN'T SOMETIMES, THIS IS ALWAYS

Jack Hall's Right Shoe

In the middle of the *Godfather III* shoot in Rome, I gave Al an ultimatum: Marry me, or at least commit to the possibility. We broke up, got back together, and went on to spend another year implementing our predictable pattern of breakups. Poor Al, he never wanted it. Poor me, I never stopped insisting. Thinking back on my motives makes me wonder why the rewards of reality kept losing out to the lure of fantasy.

When I look back on my failed romances, I invariably return to the memory of Jack and Dorothy dancing on a hill in Ensenada. Mom kept her mouth shut on the subject of marriage. Maybe she was afraid of revealing the dark side. We never discussed men, or what to expect from them, or how to grapple with disappointment. How could Mother offer up such advice when her own perception of men—I've now learned—was nothing if not muddled with contradictions? How could she bring up questions she had no answers for?

I don't know what she was protecting. Romance maybe, but not love; not real day-to-day ordinary love with its ups and downs and compromises and demands and shortcomings. I have no idea what she thought of Warren and Al. Or of me with them. She adored Woody. He took a real interest in her creative endeavors, especially photography. As for Dad, when I asked him what he thought about men he would say, "Women love bums." That's all he could come up with.

Godfather III had a lackluster, middle-aged feel. Everyone was older but not happier. Francis Coppola preferred to direct from the Silver Bullet, his trailer. Things picked up the day Winona Ryder arrived—with her fiancé, Johnny Depp— to play Kay and Michael's daughter. Winona was rushed into the makeup trailer while we were shooting. Her tiny head looked lost in the black wig the hairdresser tried to adjust. It was almost like reliving the blond wig with Dick Smith when I was twenty-three. That evening Francis was notified Winona had collapsed, which gave him the opportunity to put his daughter, Sofia, into the role of Mary Corleone. Francis told us he had written the role for Sofia in the first place.

When word got to Paramount's CEO Frank Mancuso and Sid Gannis, his Number Two, we were told they would "handle it."

The next day, "Two" flew to Palermo. At dinner, Gannis confided to Al his concerns about the Sofia Problem. Paramount didn't want her. He, Sid Gannis, was personally going to have a no-nonsense chat with Ellie, Francis's wife. Ellie? What about Francis? Needless to say, Gannis left a few days later and Sofia played my daughter, Mary Corleone.

On our way back to the hotel, Al's phone rang. Robin was on the line. It was Dad. He was acting confused. He couldn't remember Randy's name. He forgot his wallet and he wasn't even concerned. It was so not Dad. When I called a few days later, Mom told me a biopsy had revealed a stage-four glioma the size of a grapefruit lodged in his frontal lobe. She put him on the phone and I asked how he was doing. "They're going to put a brace on my head until they come across the growth. It's swollen. I have a tumor on my mind, or rather, a tumor in my brain. One of them. They tell me I'll be sitting in a class. I'll be in a program. They say they're going to radiate me. I don't know, Di-annie, I don't know. When I turned sixty-eight it all went to hell."

In a magnanimous gesture, Francis insisted I catch the next plane to L.A. When the 747 landed, I drove to UCLA Medical Center, where I found Dad looking the same, except for the bandage covering the top of his shaved head and the plastic tube filled with fluid that was attached to his arm like a leash. It made me think of the bird feeders you buy at

Builders Emporium. He was pulling his pants up, while the television set hanging from the ceiling played his favorite show, *Major Dad*. I asked him how he felt. "Oh, I've lived long enough. Sixty-eight years is plenty, Di-annie."

Dad was given a treatment option: In conjunction with radiation, he could also become part of an experimental program led by a well-known UCLA doctor, who told us Dad was a ripe candidate at the right age. His cancer was fast-acting and very invasive, but he was healthy in every other respect. His doctor at UCLA felt he was a good choice for the new treatment. Robin called it the "immunvert" stimulation of the immune system or something like that. Dad decided to give the double whammy a try. Loaded with pills, Mom drove him home to get a few things before they checked in to the Royal Palace Motel in Westwood and he began radiation.

Dr. Copeland, Dad's internist and old friend, had a different take. "It's bad. The older the age, the more aggressive the tumor. The frontal lobe controls our ability to concentrate. The likelihood? No matter what therapy he agrees to, Jack will decline. He'll lose his appetite. He'll sleep more. He'll become less active, more confused, and more disoriented. Eventually he will slip into a coma. His heart will stop, or he'll get pneumonia and die. It's a bad tumor."

Outside the Royal Palace, I took Dad's hand and walked with him to Arby's for a roast beef sandwich. I helped him take off his jacket. It was hot. My hand brushed up against a label on the inside of the collar, hand-printed in black ink. "Jack Hall's jacket. Return to 2625 Cove St., Corona del Mar, California." Dad was a stickler about identifying personal items. Jack Hall's robe, Jack Hall's boxer shorts, Jack Hall's pajama bottoms.

After we ate on plastic chairs drilled into the floor, we sauntered back to the Palace, a mid-sixties structure with a large neon sign welcoming travelers to its royal warmth. It looked harmless enough, but inside, it quickly revealed its true colors. Hairless men and gaunt women sat under the glare of the fluorescent-lit lobby. Defeat permeated the atmosphere. Everyone looked like boarders on borrowed time. Mom and Dad's little suite didn't make me feel better. I saw a pair of Dad's loafers next to the bed. Jack Hall's left shoe. Jack Hall's right shoe.

The Big Machine

The next day Dad and I wandered through UCLA's massive complex until we reached the radiation room. It was dark, maybe to soften the look of the afflicted. "Well, I guess it's time for the guy who does the camera work down in the dungeon to take the big picture. If he keeps zapping me in the head, I'm going to look like Yul Brynner." Sitting down, I looked over and saw Rocco Lampone, the button man, from *The Godfather*. What was he doing here? Tom Rosqui, aka Rocco Lampone, came over to say hello. He wanted to know about *Godfather III*. He was sorry he'd been killed off in *II*. When the loudspeaker called Jack Hall's name, Tom suddenly clasped my hand. He was getting radiation too. As I steered Dad into the room with the big machine, Tom waved goodbye. He died the following year. Radiotherapy didn't help him, not for very long; longer than Dad, but not long enough.

The X-ray machine, a sickly beige, was at least twenty years old. It looked like a massive appliance from the fifties—a sort of toaster, grill, and steamer room rolled into one. The attendant marked Dad's head with green X's, designating the areas to be radiated. The machine, exhausted after battling cancer for so long, seemed harmless. After Dad was strapped onto the gurney, I watched the shadow of his head move across a floor-to-ceiling photo mural of giant redwoods.

On the way back to the Royal Palace, Dad and I walked down Le Conte Avenue, past the old Bullock's parking lot. He wasn't in a hurry. Holding my hand in the midday heat, he stopped and looked at the ground for a while, then looked some more. Bending down, he picked up a plastic ring and gave it to me.

Dad had taken to contemplating the design of things like broken pencils, dents on tables, and even the configuration of drops of water in the kitchen sink. The boundaries of what was considered worthy of his curiosity had expanded, like the universe. As I put the Cracker Jack prize on my little finger, Dad wandered off to become friends with a giant sycamore tree's temporary tenant, a robin redbreast.

That night we went to dinner at Plum West. Mom wore a black dress, topped off with a pair of Dad's red plaid boxer shorts wrapped around her neck like a scarf. He was her man. She had his underwear on to prove it. Dad ate all his moo shu pork and drank his Johnnie Walker Red on the rocks. We were happy. It was as if we'd always be happy. Of course it wasn't true, but what lasts longer—the truth, or the memory of a perception of happiness? I opened my fortune cookie. "Value what you have now, so as not to miss it when it's gone."

After two weeks of radiation, Dad said, "I feel like I'm brain-dead. It's interesting, Di-annie; I don't know where I am half the time. I feel pretty good except when they stick their fingers up my ass every day." After two weeks Dad's head was crispy. He didn't complain, but he did say things like "I woke up in the middle of the night. I wanted to brush the hair out of my head before it cracks. I started looking for the brush but couldn't find it. I figured I'd put Dorothy on the case. But when she opened the refrigerator, there was a pigeon inside looking for its sunglasses."

Mom was starting to lose it. "You know, I think I should drive him to Santa Monica, so he can put his feet in the sand and look at the waves. He needs it. I'm worried, Diane. They're frying him raw. And what are those pills doing to him? He doesn't say a word. He just takes it. He's going downhill fast. He orders shakes at Arby's, but I can't get him to drink them. He doesn't eat. The doctor is alarmed. But how alarmed can he be? Anyone can see that Jack's an experiment that's destined to fail? I think the 'alarm' is centered on the experiment, not Jack."

To watch my father analyze his toothbrush in the bathroom of his suite at the Palace or wait patiently with Rocco Lampone and the other cancer patients was unbearable. He would say things like "Life is transitory. We're just traveling through." And "It's like the circus, Diane: If you're going to go to the damn thing, you should see it all the way through."

After another couple of weeks Dad's head was red, as red as a robin redbreast, brighter than a red-winged blackbird, and even brighter than the brightest of all the red cardinals.

On April 13, Dad prematurely flunked the "program" and was driven home in an ambulance to be more comfortable. "It's the quality of life, not the quantity," his doctor told us. An air of disbelief prevailed. He might get better. Right? At the same time, Dad was looking more wounded. His failure to live up to the program's requirements was obvious.

It was the afternoon of Christ's ascension when Dad dispersed six legal pads in front of six chairs surrounding the dining room table, and it was the last time the entire Hall family would gather together. He passed around six pencils and presented what looked to be a thickly bound notebook, sealed with dozens of rubber bands. We looked at his chronicle of financial accomplishments, including the evaluation of the estate, the estimate of the property taxes, the holdings in real estate—in short, the net worth of Jack Newton Ignatius Hall. He informed us the estate taxes would amount to approximately 55 percent. We nodded in unison. "I want to talk to you kids about the living trust and how to brace yourselves for the future." He picked up one of the yellow pencils and held it to the light of the sun. He ran his fingers across each crease. It was almost as if the pencil knew secrets. Slowly (what was the hurry?), Dad put the pencil down, rolled it across the table, then rolled it again, and again, and again. "Any questions? Randy?" Randy shook his head. "Randy, any questions?" Randy's face froze in the smile he always wore when Dad confronted him. And that was it.

Randy got up and left. Our meeting adjourned without so much as another word.

We ate lunch on the patio while Dad faced the ocean without his Johnnie Walker Red. Robin told Mom to be prepared for possible seizures. She itemized her own to-do list just in case. "Turn him on the side so he can't swallow his tongue. Don't worry, you can do it. Put your knee under his head so he can't bang it against something hard." Dad's faraway look was farther away than ever. "So much nothing, right, Dad? So much nothing, and then the big nothing."

The next time I spoke to Randy, I asked, "What happened? Why did you leave so abruptly?"

This is what he said: "I called Dad last week. After all that's gone on, I wanted him to know I loved him. You know what he said? He said, 'What's gone on?' He just couldn't go there. You know what I mean, Diane? Couldn't go there."

Dad never let go of his big plans for Randy. They were classic. John Randolph would carry on the Hall family business. Instead, he sat in his singles condo on Tangerine Street, writing poems about the journey of underground birds. Like Grammy Hall, Dad couldn't grasp it. "Birds fly, they don't live under the earth." But Randy went on to spend a lifetime writing about birds that couldn't quite take off. According to Dad, everything Randy did was ass-backward. For instance, when the temperature in the townhouse Dad bought him hit ninety degrees, Randy didn't have enough common sense to open the damn window. It drove Dad nuts. I just wished he could have understood there was no point in telling Randy what to do.

Together Again

Back in Palermo three weeks later, the tension on the set was explosive. Francis was where I left him, still sitting in the Silver Bullet, still rewriting the end. After dozens of breakups, Al and I broke up again. Masters of avoidance, we did not say hello.

It was a cold Saturday when Francis called a rehearsal in the very room where Wagner composed *Parsifal*. The usual suspects were gathered: Andy Garcia, George Hamilton, Talia Shire, Sofia (soon to be on the cover of *Vogue*), Richie Bright, Al, and John Savage. Eli Wallach came up to me. "You're a survivor. Good for you. You're a bright survivor." Survivor? The lights had been hung upside down in the Teatro Massimo. Gordon Willis was fuming. As we waited for the twelfth rewrite of the ending to *Godfather III,* I thought about the other versions. There was one where Talia kills Eli Wallach, Al is blinded, and Andy breaks off with Sofia the instant before she is assassinated. After blind Al discovers his dead daughter on the steps of the theater, he blows his brains out. There was the one where Al is assumed dead but comes back. There was the one where he is shot but lives, only to be killed on Easter Sunday on his way to church. There was the version where Al is gunned down at Teatro Massimo but Sofia lives. None of us knew what to expect. Would this be the final, final draft or just one in a continuing series of attempts to end the saga of our erratic and entirely brilliant leader Francis Coppola?

All I remember about shooting the actual final scene to *The Godfather: Part III* is this: It was easy to sob. I sobbed and sobbed, then sobbed some more. It wasn't hard. All I had to do was think of Dad. When I didn't think of him, I thought of Al. We were back together, sort of.

I didn't care if it would work or not. I was happy to hear him read *Macbeth* at midnight, just to listen to the sound of his voice. He was crazy. Crazy great. It was always "Di." "Di, make me some coffee, hot and black." "Di, come sit next to me so we can talk." One night—my favorite—I listened to him tell me about being a kid on the street. He loved the fall and how the shadows amplified the broken-down brownstones. He told me the world would always be that street in the Bronx. Every beautiful thing was compared to those days, with the light shining its gold on his friends and the street. Always the street. I listened.

He hated goodbyes. He preferred to vanish as mysteriously as he appeared. Sometimes I'd wake up in the middle of the night and find him making tea or eating popcorn and plain M&Ms. He liked plain. I liked him plain. I loved him, but my love was not making me a better person. I hate to say it, but I was *not* plain. I was *too* much.

My Story of the Story of Dad's Life

Right after I got back from finishing *The Godfather: Part III*, Dad told Mom to go look for a gun to kill the neighbors. "Do I have bad breath?" he said as he peed while kneeling in his bedroom, fingering the edge of the floorboard. He was terribly thin. He could barely hold a cup. He didn't stop to look at sparrows anymore; he'd stopped walking. Dr. Copeland had been right. It was "bad."

In the beginning of August he pretty much stopped talking too. Sometimes I would sit on the corner of his hospital bed, look out the picture window, and tell him my story of the story of his life, like the time he took us all the way to San Bernardino to a place called McDonald's, where they sold hamburgers for fifteen cents and orange juice for five. Did he remember the giant red sign that said, *Self-Service System HAMBURGERS. We have sold OVER 1 million*? Did he remember the hamburger, and the sign? Did he? He smiled but didn't nod.

One afternoon I talked to Dad about all the times we drove under the Avenue 55 overpass onto the Pasadena Freeway, until we made a left at the Pacific Coast Highway. It took us all the way to Palos Verdes. Once there, he and his friend Bob Blandin checked their lobster traps before diving off the cliffs into the ocean. Palos Verdes was famous for Lloyd Wright's all-glass Wayfarers Chapel. Mom said people wanted to get married with an ocean view. I asked Dad if he remembered how every wedding was called off after a house slid down a hill one Sunday. Did he remember how we continued driving to Palos Verdes, landslide or not, and how we kept waiting for him in the backseat of our first and only woody station wagon as we ate Mom's better-than-McDonald's homemade hamburgers wrapped in tinfoil, with cheese and mayo and dill pickles too? Did he remember coming over the cliffs every weekend, singing, "Who stole the ding-dong, who stole the bell? I know who stole it, Dorrie Bell." Did he remember how he'd always lean down to kiss little Robin Redbreast, then me, his Di-annie Oh Hall-ie? Dad tilted his head back and forth, trying to think it through. It was an awful lot of questions for a dying man to answer.

I told him the story about the time I spied on him through the crack of his bedroom door as he slipped coins into nickel-, dime-, and quarter-size candy-striped wrappers he got from the Bank of America. After he filled them, he opened a drawer and put the new wrappers on top of a mound of others. Seeing the outline of his profile as he reflected on the cumulative results of his undertaking made me smile. There he was, Mary Alice Hall's son, happily engaged in realizing a portion of his dream, the acquisition of money. I told Dad I wanted him to be sure and be proud of all the other dreams he'd realized too, big dreams, dreams he never thought he could have accomplished. I told him I hoped to pass on the memory of his accomplishments to a child of my own someday, even though I knew I was a little long in the tooth. Dad didn't respond. After that, I didn't tell him any more stories.

The fat man in the black suit came from the coroner's office. He put on rubber gloves to examine the body. It was brief. He wrapped a wire tag around my father's big toe. No more Jack Hall's right shoe, Jack Hall's left shoe. Robin, Dorrie, and I went outside and sat on the Jacuzzi cover. I looked through Dad's picture window as two men from the Neptune Society strapped him onto a gurney. Covered in a royal-blue cloth, Dad was rolled out of the living room, through the kitchen, into the garage, out the garage door, and onto the driveway. I followed the little procession from a distance. After they shut the windowed door to the van, all I could make out was the royal-blue blanket stretched across my father's body. At least he was wrapped in the color of the ocean at sunset.

What Remains

Two months after Dad died, Al admitted in the safety of the therapist's office what I must have always known: He never had any intention of marrying me. What he wanted was out. And that's what he got. He got out. I watched him walk into the light of the California sun without so much as a glance back. Later the same day, he flew to the safety of New York, the George Washington Bridge, his driver, Luke, and his dog, Lucky, waiting at Snedens Landing.

This is what remains of Al Pacino.

1. Eight pink slips from the Shangri-La Hotel in 1987, saying, "Call from Al."

2. A page ripped out of a book with the sheet music to "All I Have to Do Is Dream," inscribed "To Di" at the top of the page, "Love Al" at the bottom.

3. One happy-birthday note card, with "Love Al" written on it.

4. A handwritten letter from December 1989: "Dear Di, I am feeling uncomfortably lonely more than I have in many, many moons. I don't know why this is so. It's perhaps being in a foreign country and not being able to speak the language; you could say that's one of the reasons. But mainly it's being away from you and what we have together. As I'm

writing this letter I'm sitting in an outside café in Rome, it's pouring rain. I'm looking onto a beautiful square with a church talking to myself. I've got my hands folded as if in prayer. But in the middle of my hands is a little tape recorder. So it looks like I'm talking to my fingers. That's the way it looks. If only I could dictate this letter without moving my lips. Just trying to tell you I miss you, 'darlin'. In a sort of roundabout way it seems. I will get back to you. Love, Al."

5. A note on a torn piece of paper: "Diane, Andy, me, and Don went to a restaurant in Mondello. I will call you with the name of the joint. Sit tight be right. Don't fight. Love Al, Your friend."

6. January 29, 1992, handwritten: "Dear Di. I heard that Anna Strasberg talked to you on the phone and may have mentioned something about my sending regards or some such amenity. Never did I do that. I would never use such a coy approach to trying to communicate with you. It's unbearable to think that you would get that impression. I need no go between if I want to contact you. I apologize for having put you through this note. L. Al Pacino."

7. August 19, 1995, on Chal stationery, typed: "Dear Di, Thank you for your very beautiful note about Lucky. Your warm words, thoughts, and deep understanding of my relationship with Lucky made me feel not alone. Thank you. Meanwhile, I heard about your mother and the news was upsetting to me. I send to you my thoughts and hopes for her recovery. I know it's very difficult. It's seriously a hard life, and that's all there is to it. I feel now, of course, helpless to do anything for you except to let you know that I have some understanding for what you're going through. Once again,

thank you for your note. It helped me. My thoughts are with you, and I think about you often. Love, Al."

A Portrait

At the end of November, Dad's remains sat on the bookshelf of our Tubac, Arizona, home. Dorrie and Mom were waiting. I was flying in from Dallas to join them. Early that morning, Dorrie woke to the sound of a thud. She opened the sliding glass door to find a mourning dove lying in a pool of blood.

I arrived in time to help finish making Dad's cross. We three women walked to the top of the little incline overlooking the valley below the Santa Rita mountain range. We hammered the handmade wooden cross into the ground. We thumbtacked a photograph of Dad above his name, date of birth, and date of death. We stuck a couple of hundred-dollar bills underneath the rocks. We figured he'd want a little cash on his trip. We placed the mourning dove alongside Dad so he'd have a traveling companion. We weren't sure of their destination, but we felt better knowing he wouldn't be alone.

1990 was the year I lost my father. It was also the year I lost Al. In a way, Dad's dying was a preparation for Al's goodbye. During Dad's five short months living with brain cancer, I learned that love, all love, is a job, a great job, the best job. I learned that love is much more than a fantasy of romance. It turned out losing Al was predictable, but losing Dad was not. Losing Dad would change me in ways I never could have guessed.

One day I took a photograph of Dad looking unflinch-
ingly into the face of death. He was pretty much flying on his
own, soaring over California, checking out the lay of the
land just before he was about to make his last flight. Some
people say photographs lie. My father's eyes gazing out of
prolonged suffering is the truth to me. I'm aware that it
might seem peculiar to focus on a portrait of dying Dad
rather than young Dad or dynamic Dad. Yet I can't pass it
without reflecting on the way he left. Stripped of reason, hal-
lucinating dogs doing backflips in his bedroom, Dad was on
a wild ride. His face in his sixty-eighth year makes me hope
I can engage in life the same way he engaged death. Straightforward, unembellished, and uncluttered.

"I know I can't take this world with me. I don't even
know where I am half the time, but I'll tell you, Diane, I feel
better. You never realize how much you appreciate the little
things. Your Mudd, for instance. I love your mother, even
though I never know what she's going to do." It wasn't Norman Vincent Peale. It wasn't Dale Carnegie. What it was was
Dad.

11
AFTERMATH

Two Letters

Dear Dad,

It's the first day of 1991. I think you would have been happy to see your girls today. The sun shone through a dense marine layer at 10. Robin went to the store towing Riley and little Jack, now a toddler. Dorrie, Mom, and I went to look at an open house on Ocean Drive. Can you believe they were asking 2.5 million dollars for a 2,000 square foot box with a marginal view? You would have been proud of Mom. She nearly gagged.

Back at Cove St., Dorrie put on Willie Nelson. I opened a bottle of wine, and we all sat down to one of Mom's delicious tuna casseroles. The kids ate candy for dessert, your favorite, See's chocolate turtles.

It was unseasonably hot, so Robin, Dorrie, and I
swam over to Big Corona, where we caught waves with
people who don't own homes on the beach. Thank you
for our little box with a view, Dad. When Mom and the
kids joined us we built sand castles. Riley taught me
how to make them correctly. She'll end up in management. She's your kind of girl. Little Jack bent over a collection of buckets on the shoreline, examining sand
crabs.

I think you would have gotten a big kick out of
your three daughters eyeing all the hunks. Dorrie
joked about my type. I want to reiterate: I don't have
a type, Dad. I know you think all women love bums,
but you're wrong. It's complex. Al and I broke up a
couple of months after you died. It's been sad, but
educational. I wonder if I'll ever find a better way to
love a man, the "correct" way. I wish you and I had
been closer. I wish I'd been a Daddy's girl. Your girl.
I wish I had figured out a way to love you with a little
less effort.

In any event it was a good day, this first day of
1991. We were happy at the beach. It was just us, your
five girls, and a little boy named after you. Jack.
Love, Diane

Dear Jack,

*I want to talk to you about some things I regret I've
learned too late. I know you wouldn't want me to live
with regrets. And I'm trying not to, but I look at
couples bickering about some small matter and I want*

to say, "Don't take your living time fighting & fussing over nothing. Be happy. You have one another."

I still feel your presence. When that feeling comes I look up to the sky (as if that's where you are), and I think if I feel you so intensely you must have a sense of me also. If that's true you know that I am feeling old. I hate to confront the fact that I'm slipping in my mental capacities too. It bothers me. I still have the red heart you gave me last Valentine's Day full of See's chocolates. Or was that the year before? Oh, God, Jack, you see what I mean. It's all slipping away.

I would like to request a favor from you. Please be with me, for I am very much in need of you. Force your way through to me, will you? Please. I am lonely. I don't know why it was so hard for me to tell you how much I loved you when you were sitting across from me on the bar stool, drink in hand, music playing, dinner cooking, all things working. Maybe you know all the answers now that you've gone to the other side. All I know is I held you in my arms as you lay dying. I want to go that way too. But who will hold me, Jack? Who will hold me now that you've gone?

I love you.

Your Dorothy

The Price of Pretty, March 1991

It's funny how the rain came so suddenly. A mud slide crushed the yellow crocuses in my backyard. Even at dinner

with Dana Delany and Lydia Woodward, two fantastic single gals, my mind was never far from the avalanche. Dana
ordered a glass of cabernet. She wanted to know if I was dating. I mentioned a guy in Newport Beach. "Did he do you?"
Dana asked. "No," I said. "No, he did not do me." I hadn't
been done.

What I wanted to say was, my lungs were filled with a
residue of dust from the past. Why did I have to be intrigued
by the Goth with bloody cuts decorating his tattooed neck
outside Musso and Frank instead of the happy-faced family
eating vanilla ice cream as they entered the Hollywood Wax
Museum? Why was Lydia's loneliness more compelling than
Dana's conquests and confidence?

After Al, I lost all semblance of Dana's sexy confidence.
The truth is I never had it, but that isn't the point. The point
is I let myself, yet again, become preoccupied with failure.
Mine. Maybe I wasn't pretty enough for Al. Maybe Al, like
Ronnie McNeeley back in junior high, wasn't attracted to
my face. My face was my failure.

Sometimes it's hard to separate the concept of beauty
from the concept of pretty. They're different. Beauty is vari-
able. It comes and goes. For example, Grammy Hall was
beautiful once and only once, and that was the year she died.
Natalie Wood went from pretty to beautiful in *Splendor in
the Grass*. Anna Magnani was an ugly beauty who flung herself onto the dirt in *Rome, Open City*. All these women were
beautiful. They were mesmerizing, but their beauty didn't
make promises. It wasn't safe, and it wasn't eternal.

If I wanted to be pretty I could put in an order for a
face-lift, with an eye job on the side, and I could get rid of

my Irish bulb to boot. Plastic surgeons would be happy to accommodate my needs. But then what? It's a little late to start experimenting. And besides, pretty, with its promise of perfection, is not as appealing as it used to be. What is perfection, anyway? It's the death of creativity, that's what I think, while change, on the other hand, is the cornerstone of new ideas. God knows, I want new ideas and new experiences.

The difference between prettiness and beauty is that prettiness—like the Avon lady knocking at your door, offering up a selection of neatly wrapped gratification—is a dead end. Beauty, flinging itself onto the earth like Anna Magnani, is alive and fleeting. I'd like to let go of pretty with no hard feelings, but do I have it in me? Beauty is not an option. Beauty is like living with questions. There are no answers. If beauty is in the eye of the beholder, does that mean mirrors are a waste of time? I don't know if I'm brave enough to live without answers or to stop looking at myself.

Life Goes On

HBO offered me the role of Hedda Nussbaum, a victim of domestic abuse whose adopted daughter, Lisa, died from a severe blow to the head given by Joel Steinberg, Hedda's lover. I passed. No more victims for me. Instead, I restored the Wright house Dad had warned me not to buy. I took a road trip to Canyon de Chelly with Dorrie. I directed a music video called "Heaven Is a Place on Earth" with Belinda Carlisle. I took a screenwriting class at USC with

David Howard, who talked about preparation and aftermath. "You're never too old to learn, huh?" a student asked during a break. "Yeah, never too old," I said. I met a producer named Judy Polone, who gave me a shot at directing a TV movie called *Wildflower.* We hired the cinematographer Janusz Kaminski, who went on to shoot *Schindler's List* for Steven Spielberg. I cast Patricia Arquette and Reese Witherspoon to star. They were beautiful and talented. The future was theirs. Randy moved to Laguna. Al had a baby. Warren married Annette Bening. Dorrie bought a house. Robin had two children, one husband, and three rescue dogs. I kept moving.

At the Rose Bowl swap meet, Carolyn Cole, the director of the Los Angeles *Herald Examiner* photography collection at the Los Angeles Central Library, came up to me and wanted to know if I was interested in taking a look at something very special. Alone in the basement of Bertram Goodhue's Egyptian revival landmark, I opened the file marked *A* and began a trip through two million photographs of found dogs, missing children, holdup suspects, wife beaters, crossdressers—basically the whole kitchen sink of down-and-outers who shared a short-lived if splashy notoriety in the *Herald Examiner.* I found an eight-by-ten picture of Mother Anderson, who had been caught passing bad checks at Clifton's Cafeteria while pregnant with her seventeenth child. Behind her was a photograph of Father Anderson in jail, accused of kidnapping one of their daughters. Blind ex-G.I. Edward Altman was pictured reunited with his Seeing Eye dog, Trump, and Gladis Archer was photographed in pants after she was freed from jail for having worn a Marine uniform to a drinking party. Subscribers like Grammy Hall and George Olsen ate up the insatiable black hole of someone else's misfortune.

In the *A*'s, under "The Ambassador Hotel," I found a picture of triumphant Dorothy Hall being crowned Mrs. Los Angeles by Art Linkletter. But under "Abandoned," there was no photograph of Beulah Keaton scrubbing toilets at Franklin High School in her new occupation as janitor. What about her hard-luck story? The story of a woman who woke up to see her husband of twenty-five years drive off to Utah in the family's only car with a woman he was about to marry, thus becoming a bigamist. There was no picture of little Jackie Hall's face pressed against a window as he watched his mother, Mary Alice, play blackjack inside one of Catalina Island's notorious gambling ships at one A.M. In fact, there were no stories or pictures of the other Halls or Keatons. For me, the thin line between newsworthy and not was converging. A book began to take shape. A kind of tabloid family of man. I called it *Local News*.

When Woody asked me to fill in for Mia Farrow on *Manhattan Murder Mystery*, I took the job. It was crazy. Outside, the press circled Woody's trailer. A day didn't go by without microphones in his face. "What's your take on the custody battle with Mia Farrow?" Inside, it felt like *Annie Hall* days, only looser, if that was possible. Carlo Di Palma shot the movie handheld. Entire scenes were completed in one take. We were in makeup at seven A.M. and wrapped at two-thirty in the afternoon. I couldn't believe how easy it was. As for Woody, he never brought up personal problems while working.

Unstrung Heroes

Donna Roth and Susan Arnold were looking for a director. *Unstrung Heroes* was based on Franz Lidz's memoir about the struggle of a boy named Steven after his mother, Selma, is diagnosed with ovarian cancer. When Selma begins to fade, Steven's father has him stay with his two uncles, one a hoarder, the other a paranoid. They teach him to value his own uniqueness. Uncle Arthur in particular gives Steven a way of appreciating the beauty found in mundane objects like string and rubber balls. But it's Selma who gives him the capacity to love. Steven creates his own memorial to Selma before she dies by filling a box with her things—a tube of her lipstick, a perfume bottle, a cigarette lighter.

Finding redemption through documentation was particularly moving to me. It was almost as if Franz Lidz was telling us that items, possessions, even stuff, could make up for the mercurial comings and goings of love. I auditioned with Donna and Susan by giving them my thoughts, particularly those related to documenting a family's history. I'd been mimicking Mom for years by writing my own journal. The subject was personal. Susan and Donna were the kind of producers who had enough confidence to give me a try.

It was my first feature as a director. I needed help in every department. I hired a USC film graduate, Greg Yaitanes, as the visual consultant. He had an imaginative approach and was highly inventive with action. Together we shot the film before I shot the film. It may seem insane, but Greg operated the videocam while I played dying Selma, young Steven, even

The secret is still in the family.
And you share it eve...

SOL
N G

II
RA

II
W

You ca
Every
"Ma

Y

Honor thy self.

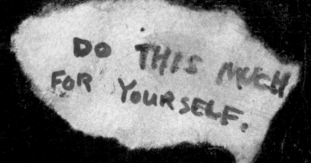

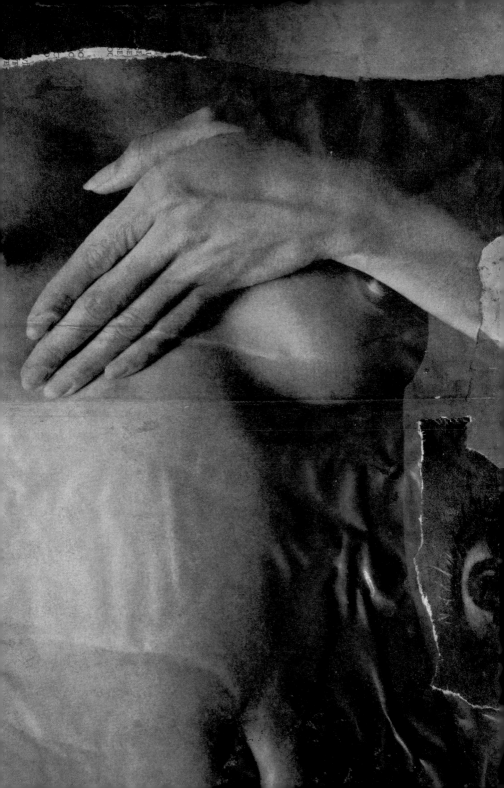

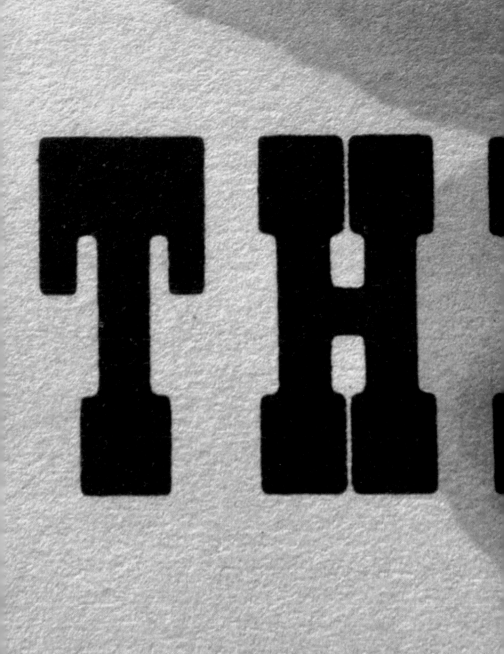

INK

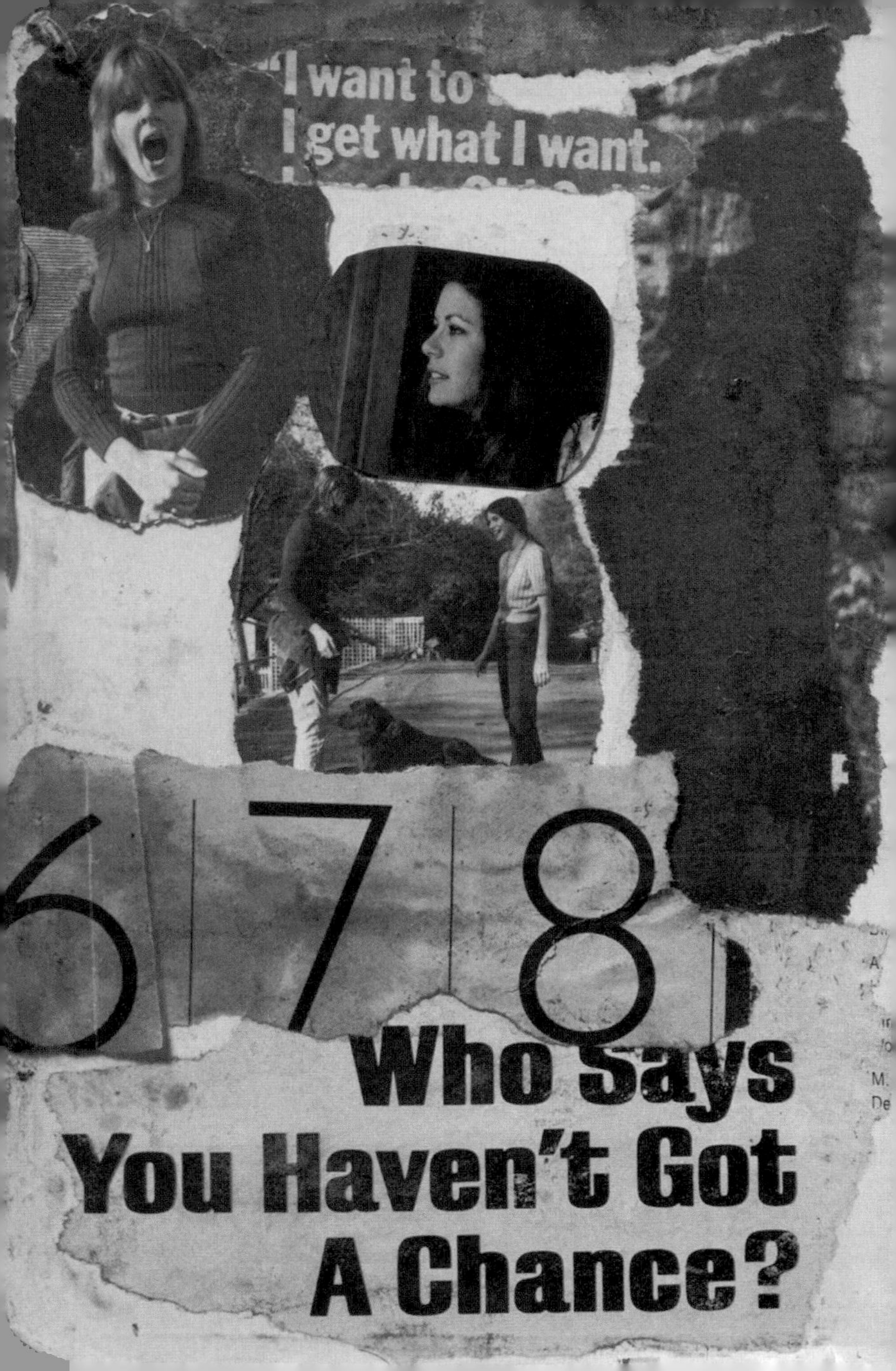
"I want to
I get what I want.
6 7 8
Who Says
You Haven't Got
A Chance?

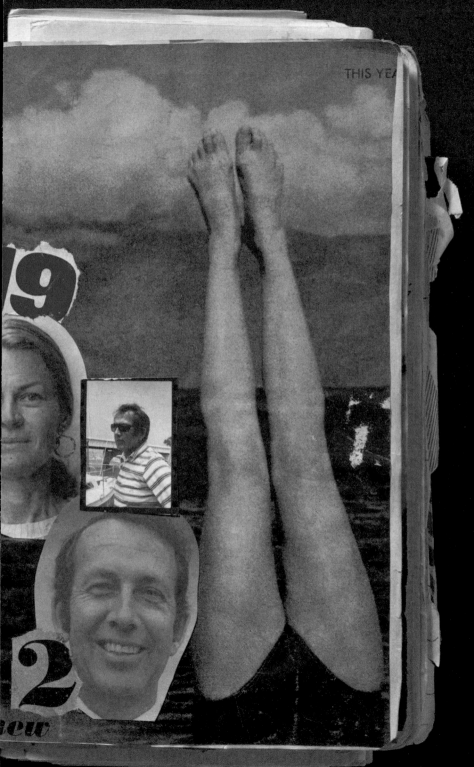

I CAN'T GET ANY FEELINGS ABOUT WRITING IN THIS......

or not to be

crazy Uncle Danny. Speaking their words made me feel more connected to the story. When we started principal photography, I was grateful I had my little video movie of the movie to help with camera setups. Phedon Papamichael, our cinematographer, went along with my folly. In fact, all department heads were willing to go along with my so-called "vision." The music, composed by Tom Newman, was nominated for an Academy Award. Garreth Stover, the production designer, was full of ideas. Bill Robinson, my soon-to-be partner, was invaluable. All the actors broke my heart. Andie MacDowell, lovely Andie; the late Maury Chaykin, a great actor and friend; Michael Richards, the reason Disney green-lit the film; John Turturro; and quirky little Nathan Watt were unique, idiosyncratic, singular, and wonderful. I loved them all. I wish I had made a better movie. Having directed two feature films, I'm more acutely aware of how nearly impossible it is to make a good film.

When *Unstrung* was selected for Un Certain Regard at the Cannes Film Festival, Disney flew me over. Susan Arnold told me not to worry: The plane was safe, we'd have a great flight, we would drink red wine. I took a Xanax instead. Once I was there, Cannes was a spectacular scene. My interviews with Kevin Thomas of the *Los Angeles Times,* E! Entertainment, HBO, the Toronto *Star, Time* magazine, and CNN were positive. Joe Roth, the head of Disney, wanted to know what my next picture was going to be. At the party, Richard Corliss's wife talked about the theme of hands, how delicately the hands stood out in scene after scene. Wanting to end on a high note, I slipped into the official Cannes limo and disappeared into the dead of night. Inside my suite at

the Carlton, a familiar sensation came back. With my Miz-
rahi dress in the closet, the party was over. I was alone
again—this time in Cannes. It wasn't different from any
other night, except I didn't have my dog, Josie, to pet, which,
as lame as it may seem, gave me something to look forward
to. Just the thought of stroking her mangy coat, grabbing
her muzzle, and laying on lots of kisses made me feel good. I
missed the ritual, the every-night of it, the knowing she'd be
there. How was it possible that Josie—the shepherd mix who
bit the mailman and attacked the neighbor's dog, Freddy;
Josie, aka Jaws, the dog I wouldn't have wished on anyone—
was the only thing I missed as I stared at the ceiling in a
beautiful hotel suite six thousand miles away from my very
own "yellow snapper"?

Diane's Journal, May 29, 1995

With eight hours left on the twelve-hour flight, the *Fasten
Your Seat Belt* sign goes on for the fifth time. I start to grip
the arms of the seat. It isn't like I haven't been warned. The
storm clouds at the airport were impossible to overlook. At
the ticket counter a woman in a straw hat complained to her
husband about plane connections in Las Vegas. What about
taking off in a storm, lady? I tried to distract myself with
Time magazine's profile of Reynolds Price, whose new book,
The Promise of Rest, had "rounded off a powerful saga of
isolation." Isolation. Did I have to be reminded I was flying
alone? Where was Warren to hold my hand? I thought of
Dad. He, too, found air travel intolerable. Did he feel iso-

lated in the sky? When the plane was delayed I read "Heart-break Motel," an article singling out the leftover lives of drifters, boozers, and itinerant families found in motels along the Arizona border, as lightning lit the sky. There was Paul Coyle, who, after his wife left him, had the names of his sixteen children in a heart tattooed on his back. Another tattoo read I LOVE MY FAMILY. MARRIED OCT. 12, 1958, CITY TEMPLE, ILL. PAUL AND JANET COYLE. He must have figured if he died his family would find him. One thing I knew, there'd be no family finding me if, God forbid, the delayed Boeing 747 nonstop to L.A. crashed over the Atlantic Ocean.

I hate the *Fasten Your Seat Belt* sign. I hate it. Bouncing around at 35,000 feet is just plain horrifying. Plus, the two Xanax and the glass of wine have failed. Like a car shifting from fourth to third gear, the sound of the motor, at least to me, indicates the plane is trying to adjust to a lower altitude. Is this a good idea? Isn't higher smoother? The stewardess tries to convince me everything is all right, but the thousand-foot drops are killing me. I imagine our jumbo jet flipping over upside down. I can see my face smashed against the window. When she launches into the old "car on a bumpy road" analogy, I wonder if she's crazy. She can't be serious. This is not a bumpy road. This is the air. This is being in the middle of nothing with nothing to hold on to. Sorry, but check it out. Flying is not normal. And guess what? I don't care where we are, can we please ask the captain to please make it smooth, or something? Anything. Land it some-where, I don't know, England, or how about Barbados? Whatever landmass we're near. I don't care. Anything. I can't take it anymore.

The *Fasten Your Seat Belt* light goes out. On cue my heart stops pounding. I start in with the usual promises of change. I'll spend more time with Mom. I'll stop with the endless projects and the half-assed solutions to a meaningful life.

It reminds me of the day I drove Dad home from UCLA's Medical Center after he flunked "The Program." I remember all those placating words the doctors and their staff used during Dad's two-month stay, but especially "It's the quality of life, not the quantity." Dad didn't look like a man with much quality left. We were silent as we headed south on the 405. The traffic was slow. I didn't know what to say. Two blocks before Cove Street, two blocks away from Dorothy, Dad blurted out, "Diane, I want you to know something. I've always hated my work. I wish I'd traveled more, gotten closer to you kids, taken more risks." It was his use of the word *risk* that made me think of the risks I hadn't taken, especially those revolving around intimacy. It also made me think of the time Kathryn Grody told me Estelle Parsons had adopted a baby boy at age fifty. Wasn't she too old to be adopting a baby? It made me remember my sixteen-year-old pledge not to have intercourse before I was married. Boy, that would have been a big loss, particularly since I've never married. And what about the time I told Mom I was against psychiatry on principle. What principle? Where would I be without analysis? I was intolerant of everything I went on to benefit from.

As soon as I see L.A. spread out below, I know I'm going to have to reinvent the future. I know I have to make a decision that will or will not lead to the experience of a different kind of love, a love of less expectations on the receiving end. I know if I adopt a baby I will need to adapt to conditions that require care and responsibility, and management skills too. But above all I will need to earn the right to be a mother, especially considering I am a single white woman staring fifty in the face.

12

HELLO

The Bundle

Dexter came to me in a straw basket with two handles. The first thing we did was drive to the pediatrician's office. As I put her in the new car seat, she looked cautious; after all, she'd flown across the country to meet up with a woman she would have to learn to call Mother. Everything about her was new: her tiny hands and feet, her big round face. When the doctor deemed her "alert," that meant she had passed her first test. She was alert, and attentive, and prepared, and vigilant. That was the moment I knew I had it in me to take on the rest of the tests Dexter would have to pass for as long as I lived. That's when I put my hand on her face, looked into her eyes for as long as forever will ever be, and smiled. I knew I could do it. I knew the dust from the past had lifted. Yes, Warren was right, I was a late developer, but I'd become a woman, despite my protestations, and now a mother too. Dexter was my "in sickness and health, till death do us part," unconditional love. She was my new family, this sturdy, resilient, alert girl from North Carolina.

Born Thursday, December 14, 1995, Dexter flew to Houston, Texas, four days after she was born. She arrived in Los Angeles the following Friday. On Saturday, Uncle Rickey, Robin's husband, drove Dexter and me all the way to Tubac, Arizona, for Christmas with the family. Dexter was up for the frequent diaper changes at various gas stations with other fellow Americans on their way to Christmas cheer. She appeared to be content with the steady movement of the car on the road. When we arrived at Mom's ranch, Aunt Robin, Aunt Dorrie, Grammy Dorothy, Cousin Riley, Cousin Jack, and my friend Jonathan Gale gathered around Dexter in the living room. We all agreed she had a sly smile, almost as if "Prove it" would inform her character. At ten days she was unusually street-smart and ready to go.

As if that wasn't enough, two weeks later Dexter and I flew to New York so I could complete filming on *The First Wives Club,* a comedy about three old friends who are dumped by their husbands. Ivana Trump summed up the film's message best with "Ladies, you have to be strong and independent, and remember, don't get mad, get everything."

Dexter and I had a ritual. Every night after work, I placed her in the bouncy chair and marveled at her almost fishlike, slow-motion, underwater gestures. Sometimes she followed me with her eyes. Sometimes I tried to imitate her expressions, but how could I? I've lived too long to go back to the beginning. I held her against my chest. It was hard to believe she weighed less than a medium-size bowling ball. I touched her face and gave her kisses. I put the bottle in her mouth. She swallowed the formula. Simple miracles. I began to appreciate the comfort of furniture, not just the design. More simple miracles.

In the mornings at the rented loft on Prince Street, I fed her and changed her diaper. I talked to her too. There was a lot to say. Sometimes, not always, she'd crack a smile. Then came the most important task of the day: selecting an outfit, at least 70 percent of which were gifts. First I chose one of Dexter's twenty-two hats, thirteen of which came from Kate Capshaw. Then I'd pause for a moment and go over the list of people who'd been so generous. There was Woody Allen, who gave her a flowery little dress I returned. (Too small.) Meryl Streep gave Dexter four boxes of dresses, and hats (more hats) and blankets, and jumpers and leggings and tops, and washcloths that she called a starter kit. Bette Midler gave her a health book and a very funny carrot hat with a pea on top. Then my boss, Mr. Scott Rudin, gave Dexter a fancy French coat from a store called Bonpoint on Madison Avenue. Steve Martin gave her a much needed and very practical diaper bag. Martin Short and his lovely bride, Nancy, sent her flowers and balloons that flew up to the ceiling and stayed there for two weeks. I could not believe our good fortune—a once-in-a-lifetime complete wardrobe from a host of remarkable notables.

First Ladies

Always on the go, Dexter and I went out to dinner three times a week. She came to the set every day. We took the Circle Line and saw the Statue of Liberty during a snowstorm. Bill Robinson, who'd been an intern for Ted Kennedy, made arrangements for a tour of the White House. Veteran travelers, we grabbed the first train to Washington, D.C.

We began our visit in the Oval Office. It was very yellow and blue—official blue. We took pictures in the pressroom— beside a surprisingly antiquated phone system underneath a wall of tiny black-and-white television sets monitoring the whereabouts of the First Family. The phone system was obsolete, and the television sets were tiny. In the East Room, where Presidents John F. Kennedy and Abraham Lincoln had lain in repose before burial, Dexter dozed off in her BabyBjörn. When we moved on to the Red Room, I learned Eleanor Roosevelt had changed it from a ladies' social setting to a pressroom for women reporters who were excluded from presidential conferences. The stipulation? Mrs. Roosevelt's press conferences were limited to subjects centered on "women's work."

Every office had a gadget called "the toaster." Like the monitors, its function was to inform the employees of the exact whereabouts of the President, the First Lady, Chelsea, and Socks, their cat. We were told that Hillary and Chelsea were actually in the White House. Chelsea was watching a movie, and Hillary was upstairs with a cold. She, of course, wanted to meet us but was feeling under the weather. Frankly, if I were her, I would cherish every moment of privacy and guard it like a treasure. Her life was nothing if not an intrusion. Imagine always being on view, always being groomed, always being judged and criticized. The more I saw, the more impossible it was to imagine the White House as a home. But then, I guess the idea of home is something you have to create for yourself.

There were many spectacular aspects to the White House, but the role of First Lady was not one of them. Even though she carries the burden of presenting the quintessential "American" family to the public, as well as rallying behind her favorite charities, visiting schools, hosting parties for traveling dignitaries, and privately advising her husband on the state of the union—all of it under the scrutiny of an entire nation—it's not considered a job and she's not paid.

We stood in front of the official First Lady portraits and listened to the guide tell us each woman was given the right to choose her own artist. A right? Who else was going to choose? I learned Eleanor Roosevelt felt she was so homely, she insisted that Douglas Chandor's portrait focus on her finest feature, her hands. The upper part of the painting was a typical portrait, until it bled into a kind of second painting, devoted to a series of monotone inserts of Mrs. Roosevelt's hands knitting and holding glasses—in short, engaged in the completion of domestic tasks. This was the same woman who, in 1948, was touted as a running mate for Harry Truman. Even Eleanor Roosevelt had to conform to the demands of a First Lady in the fourth decade of the twentieth century. Barbara Bush's newly hung painting was nothing if not predictable, until I noticed the framed portrait within the portrait of her dog, Millie—not her children or grandchildren, but Millie the dog—on the table next to her. Jackie Kennedy's was alluring in a distant, subdued sort of way. Very sixties. Nancy Reagan chose the same artist, Aaron Shikler, hoping to mirror Jackie's legacy. The difference was that Nancy, ever opposed to monochromatic colors, chose a red dress—a bright red dress. Nancy wanted to be Jackie in primary colors.

All of this goes to say what? An elite list of highly qualified unpaid women became First Ladies of the United States. What can I say? I hope Dexter will live long enough to witness all working women, including the First Lady, earning equal pay for equal work. Maybe she'll even see a portrait of a First Husband hanging on that wall.

Home Again

After viewing home life at the White House, home was on my mind. I couldn't wait to get back to Los Angeles. I was worried about Mother, whose failing memory skills were becoming more apparent. While I was in New York, she wrote a letter that became the official diagnosis of her illness.

> *Dear Diane,*
>   *Dr. Cummings told me I have the onset of ALZHEIMER'S, but I'm not buying it without further tests. I don't really know how I'll handle it, if it's true. I don't want to give up. . . . I admit I'm unable to recall names, and events sometimes, but not always. I must*

stop writing about my lapses of memory and work on recall. I have to keep trying but it "ain't easy," as Mary Hall would have said. The worst of it is people talk to me carefully. They're deferential and aware that I will undoubtedly forget something or make a mistake in judgment. I find myself unable to remember words like genes and chromosomes, nor do I know how to spell them. (It is genes.) *How do I tell my friends I have Alzheimer's? Just don't.*
Love,
Mom

In 1993 Mom had written she had Alzheimer's disease and it was "scary." But this letter two years later confirmed the inevitable. She finally understood what she hadn't remembered to admit. You see, Mom forgot to remember she was one of five million victims of the "forgetting" disease. I called Robin. Mother had just phoned her, saying she wanted to cancel her life insurance and empty out the house Dad had bought next door on Cove Street, knowing she'd eventually need help. She also said she wanted to be sure to commit suicide before she got bad. She was adamant, adding that she was going to take care of it. When I called Dorrie, she burst into tears.

Not a moment too soon, Bette Midler and Goldie Hawn and I wrapped *The First Wives Club* by dancing down the streets of New York, singing "You Don't Own Me." The next day Dexter and I flew back to California to begin our real life together. It turned out Ramon Novarro's Wright house was not suited for family living. My bedroom was the only room on the top floor. Dexter's was a closet-size space next to the living room slash kitchen on the second floor, and the office off the garage was on the first. I began looking for an authentic California Spanish hacienda.

In the meantime, Dex and I spent weekends at Cove Street. Mom adored her. She even bought a pint-size hope chest and filled it with things like puzzles and alphabet books and buckets and shovels. Dorothy was holding up. On several different occasions she had me sit down to Beulah Keaton's one and only scrapbook. In an attempt to keep memories alive, she did very well remembering her mother. It was always the same. She opened the last page first. There was Dorrie, a black-and-white fat-faced toddler, being held by gorgeous long-legged Dorothy in front of Grammy's Monterey Road clapboard bungalow. Robin stood next to them in her new glasses, while sheriff Randy shoved a toy gun into my chest. Mom always pointed out the sweet-pea vines in the background of Grammy Keaton's old backyard. I would ask if she helped plant the flowers. She would nod as she turned the pages back to an earlier time. I was becoming a more ardent observer of two phenomena: the slow beginning of life and the even slower ending under the reign of Alzheimer's' tyranny.

Dexter was eleven months when Mom held her hand at the shoreline. Jumping up and down, all excited, Dex pointed at the seagulls, saying, "Brr," like the day, like cold. "Brr." Mom, even more excited, said, "Bird, Diane. She said bird." *Bird* was Dexter's first word, or so Mom decided. I shook my head in wonder. Dexter was as happy as she had been inconsolable only hours before when her little face was all knotted up in tears. I recognized that all the love in the world cannot cushion the reality of pain. In that moment Dexter seemed knowing beyond her eleven months. It made me think of girls—little girls, teenage girls, even old girls like me—who at one point or another discover, like all girls do, their sadness.

It took a long time, but I finally bought an old Spanish house on Roxbury Drive in Beverly Hills, a Wallace Neff fixer-upper. My friend Stephen Shadley began the restoration. In the process I developed an abiding interest in all things Spanish and all things built in Los Angeles. The sheer variety, history, and magic of the classic homes of Southern California made me want to become part of an organization that successfully saved them. I joined the L.A. Conservancy and became a preservationist. Our new old home took a year and a half to restore before Dex became a little girl living in a genuine Spanish Revival house saved from demolition.

First Wives

First Wives was an unexpected hit. Bette, Goldie, and I did a ton of press. I'll never forget the conference call with Goldie and me at her home in the Pacific Palisades and Bette on the line from her loft in New York. Always a contradiction in terms, Goldie drank some awful green health concoction while she smoked. The interviewer asked, "What's better about being fifty than twenty?" Goldie plunged in with something like "Being a great mom; learning how to grow up and love yourself for who you are; coping with the discomfort of fame; loving a man by not holding on too much; letting people be who they are; helping your daughter live with the fact that her mother is famously loved by many people; getting revenge, but the right kind; learning to be spiritually aware; learning to grow into self-esteem. Those are some of the reasons why being fifty is better than being twenty." What could Bette and I add? Goldie had said it all.

"Diane, this is your mom. I hate to bother you, but I couldn't figure any way to do this. Merna down here in the Cove called and wants to know for sure when you're going to appear on TV again. If you are, let me know what day and what time. She really wants to see it, but she's bedridden. Maybe she got it wrong. I don't know. Just let me know. That'd be great. Bye bye, Diane."

Mom was beginning to leave messages on my voice mail all the time. She'd never been a phone person. The calls had a girlish aspect, as if she was concerned about things that had no relevance. I didn't consciously decide to take over her role as the family documentarian. But I began to save her messages.

Almost two years after her diagnosis, she still volunteered at the cancer thrift shop, where she put my wardrobe from *The First Wives Club* on prominent display in the window. She visited Robin in Georgia. She built a tack house for Dorrie in Tubac. She kept her friends. It's true our conversations centered on my concerns, like Dexter's oral fixations. Why did she keep sucking her dirty stuffed cow instead of a clean pacifier—which, by the way, I had doubts about too. Just the word *pacify* was not indicative of a healthy sense of self-esteem. Mom concurred while pointing out Dexter's more serious problem: eating sand. Might it have something to do with her formula? Maybe it was time to switch from Nutramigen to soy.

I began to write letters to Dexter about her development, including my concerns with her oral fixations (it takes one to know one). But there were also themes hopefully crossing the barriers of our fifty-year age gap, sort of explanations and apologies pertaining to who I am. It was my way of preserving Mother's legacy and a sense of carrying it on with my new family.

Dear Dexter, 1998

I named you Dexter Deanne Keaton for several reasons. I wanted a *D* name because of your grandmother Dorothy, your aunt Dorrie, and your mother, me, Diane. Dexter is short for dexterous, good with your hands. It also means adroit, proficient, shrewd, and wily. I gave you the middle name Deanne because your Grammy Dorothy's middle name is Deanne. I also named you Dexter because I like the sound. It has weight. I like the fun abbreviations, as in Dexie, Dex, Dext, or even DeeDee. The choice of Dexter also relates to Buster Keaton, a great clown of the silent films, and Dexter Gordon, who was an influential tenor sax jazz musician. Maybe you'll be funny. Maybe you'll love music. I hope you like your name. If you don't, you can change it later. I changed mine to Keaton because it's your grandmother's maiden name. I believe people evolve into who they want to be. In a way you create who you are.

Here's a bone of contention. More often than not, people come up to me and say, "Is that your granddaughter?" Dexter, I'm sorry I'm a Grammy-aged mother. I know it'll be a burden. But maybe you can turn it into a plus. I'm sure there will be some serious bumps on the road, but I'll try to keep up with your point of view, and I promise to listen. Maybe that way we'll find a common ground. Aunt Robin and Dorrie are considerably younger, so if anything were to happen to me they'll take care of you. I regret you don't have a father, not even a father figure, but who knows, things could and do change. I'm sorry. When I get too long in the tooth to take care of myself, I assure you I will not be a burden. You'll have your independence, just as Mother gave me mine. In return, let's cut a deal: promise me you'll be the kind of woman who has empathy for the plight of others. I'm not asking you to wear your heart on your sleeve. I'm asking you to try and put yourself in someone else's shoes and understand what it might feel like. You've been given privilege. It's a responsibility you have to live up to by being even more aware of what it's like not to be so fortunate. Stay human, sweetie, stay human.

Dexter, you're a brown-haired, brown-eyed three-year-old girl. Carol Kane says, "Ooh no, no, no, she's not a brown-haired, brown-eyed girl, Dexter's got hazel eyes and strawberry-blond hair." Kathryn Grody says you're an out-and-out blonde. Color-blind Bill

Robinson claims it's red. "She's got red hair, with green eyes." Green eyes? All I can tell you is, they're dead wrong. They want you to be their fantasy of an adorable little princess. They're making up a future you that fits their agenda. Even Mom betrayed her own sensibilities by declaring, "Dexter is a blond-haired angel." She has all kinds of theories about how special you are. Special schmeschial. I don't think this kind of encouragement is conducive to a healthy ego. Feeding you the bottomless pit of extraordinary is too much. I ought to know. Besides, what's wrong with brown hair and brown eyes? I love your chocolate orbs of impenetrable joy. All you have to do is squint them up into a smile, and the world is right. Brown is beautiful. The earth is brown. A chocolate Labrador retriever is brown. Bears are brown, and your eyes are the best brown ever. I don't want to be party to mythologizing you. Not only does it make for ridiculous expectations, it's not reality. Oh, and before I forget, one more promise. Promise me you won't be like I was, forever trying to please other people's expectations. Don't, Dex. It's a slippery slope. Brown is brown. Go with it.

Love you,

Mom

Almost Five

In the whirl of life you became three then four and almost five. All my observations remained the same but you became more and more your own person. Not my projection of who I wanted you to be, or what I thought was cute, or annoying. You've told me how much better life will be when you're five. When you're five you'll be able to ride on the roller coaster; when you're five you'll be tall enough to touch the ceiling; when you're five you'll outgrow your bed; that way you can sleep with me every night.

Meanwhile Mom is putting popcorn in the microwave for 35 minutes. Today she entered the living room with a grapefruit, asking where the kitchen is. Yesterday she had her underwear on the outside of her pants. She's long since stopped making her famous tuna casseroles. But she's fine, she says, as she wanders around the house. And for the most part she's still hanging in with a modicum of independence. The same independence you're fighting for as you approach age five. It's a backwards game when you get old, Dexter, especially for people like your grandmother, victims of an illness that reverses the order of life. As your uncle Randy says, "Her memory is walking out the back door." Anyway, hello to five, Dexter.

Dear Dexter, 2000

Along with the new millennium, there's an important subject I want to bring up. Occasionally we've talked about the addition of a brother or sister. You've expressed a modest interest in a baby sister—congratula-

tions—but not a boy. I was two when Randy came
along. He was a breeze. Then Robin came. I couldn't
stand her. Of course that changed with time, and now I
love her dearly. And Dorrie is still my adorable baby sister. Dexter, I don't know what life would be without
them. Now that I've lost my father, they're even more
invaluable; a word for you to remember. By invaluable I
mean essential, or, if not essential, then part of a quality of life that can't be replaced.

Hear me out on this; one of the big benefits of having siblings is a shared history. You will come to appreciate his or her different point of view. For example,
take the complaints you already have about me, your
tiresome mother. A sibling will help you deal with the
ups and downs of my deliberately oppressive parenting.
You will have a sounding board. He or she will help you
learn how to handle all the miscalculations and injus-
tices I will throw your way. Right? Right! Honestly,
Dex, I don't think it's a good idea for you to be an only
child. I acknowledge it's absurd for me to take on an infant at age 55; all the bottles and formulas, and diapers,
and sleepless nights. But, no matter how uncomfortable
and frustrating, or how overloaded our already highly
active lives would be, I'm thinking of making an execu-
tive decision. Imagining you at 30 and me at 80, you
know what I see? I see you won't want to be alone.
You'll wish you had a sister or brother. There's no getting around it. I think this is the right time to say hello
to one more life. One more, Dex; one more.

13

THE GRAY ZONE

January 1, 2001

I was knocking on the gray door of Mom's freshly painted gray house with the gray trim and the gray gate blocking the ocean view when Mom peeked her head out of the kitchen window. Dex and I walked into what can only be described as "erosion." Pulling open the kitchen drawer to make a couple of grilled cheese sandwiches, I found greasy silverware—the result of the plaque building barriers in Mom's brain. As always, I asked myself the same damn question. Were the tangles and twists growing on the outer edges of her cerebral cortex the cumulative effects of her lifelong insecurity? Could depression and self-doubt be a precursor to Alzheimer's? As always, it was the same answer. There is no answer.

Upstairs in her workroom, I came across what must have been her last attempt at a journal. What can I say except where did the words go? She still cut pictures, but the subject matter had changed from detailed photo collages of our family to cute kitties unraveling balls of yarn. She still thumbtacked items onto her kitchen bulletin board, like Frank Sinatra's obituary, next to the cover of an old *New Yorker* magazine with the caption "Is it possible to go backwards and forwards at the same time?"

At dusk the tide was low on the horizon. A lone blue heron stood on the rocks as the sun drifted toward an early sunset. Dex found a lavender starfish in the shallow water. She rushed to Grammy's five-foot cement seawall to share her find. Mom, still excited by the wonder of any found item, leaned over. Dexter pulled. Mom fell like a clump of solid mass, landing with a thud. It was Mom who took a dive. Not Dex. Mom with her white hair. Mom with her perplexed gaze. That was the day I learned to stop trusting her judgment calls. All of them. It was the beginning of a long string of inexplicable choices that had to be overseen by a caregiver.

Message, 2001

"Hi, Diane, this is your mom. I just want to tell you I got my . . . I got my beautiful"—big sigh—"oh, God, look at my memory. I got the things you sent. Right now, under pressure, I can't remember . . . huh, I know it sounds, uh . . . My wreath, that's it, the wreath is wonderful. . . . Okay, here it goes. So I'm all set and, uh, hope to see you soon, and thanks again. It's very nice. Thank you so much, Diane, okay, bye bye."

Two Mints Instead of One

I flew to New York on February 16, 2001, and checked in to the Plaza. My suite was on the second floor. The ceilings were high. The hallway was wide. My friends Kathryn Grody and Frederic Tuten came by at six. The knock came at seven. Two chirpy women with a basket (another basket) entered, carrying you. Wrapped in a blue blanket, a blue hat, a blue crocheted sweater, a blue print Onesie with blue mittens and blue booties; I got it, you're a boy. The basket was received with gratitude, and I picked you up. You have long, long, long fingers, and long feet with long toes, and skinny legs and skinny arms and tiny black buttons for eyes. Oh, my God, you have a cleft chin; promise me you won't become a movie star. Here you are, little big man. Dexter's brother, Junior Mint number two . . . my son.

To Duke

Dear Duke,

You're five months old. It's been a bit of a trial, considering the constant battles with that tummy of yours. Here's the lay of the land. After you knock down a whopping five ounces of formula, you burp. Within fifteen minutes four of the five ounces finds its way to the couch, the kitchen floor, your blankie, our sweaters, beds, you name it. Josie, the dog, trails behind, knowing she'll get her daily soy quota.

In the midst of this routine you're alternately un-comfortable, cranky, fidgety, sweet, and flirty. The doc-tor says you're strong in spite of your condition, which has been described as classic colic baby one day or typi-cal reflux infant another. You're intense. Your hands are sensory seekers, especially as they roam across my face. I don't know what you think you're going to find. Ev-erything about you is big except your size. You and I share many of the same traits. The difference is you're fast, a born handicapper. Dexter doesn't complain about all the attention you're getting. She likes to feed you, sometimes. She likes to give you kisses, sometimes. She's pretty stoic about our new "intrusion." She seeks solace in the thrill of her body flying through space in the Six Flags Hurricane Harbor roller coaster.

You're a very different baby than Dex was. It's al-ready clear you will communicate your needs. Some-times I worry—well, frankly, Duke, I worry all the time. Let me explain; yesterday Dexter's school called to inform me of an incident. Apparently one of her classmates, a girl, told Dexter she was born in the pound, bought at the zoo, and didn't have a real mother. Dexter's response was unfathomable. My re-sponse to her response was exactly—well, sort of— what the experts said to say. "Dex, being adopted is like finding yourself with a whole new family." Whatever that means? What I didn't say was this. Everyone is sort of adopted, in that eventually we're all abandoned in one way or another. What constitutes a family? Hard to say. Take me. I was born into an attractive-looking post–World War II family, with a daddy and mommy and three siblings. We appeared normal, but we weren't. Who is? The idea of family can be expansive, as in extended family. Duke, you have two mothers; one had the wherewithal to know she couldn't raise you given her set of circumstances. The other, me, chose to take care of you, and always will. Someday you may decide to make your own family. You might marry and have children of your own. You may even consider close friends as part of your family. These are options, and there are many more. Think Big.

Being adopted is to start life with loss. It's not necessarily a bad thing. Loss helps us learn how to handle goodbyes. Like Dexter, one day someone will tell you you're adopted, as if you are less than your typical run-of-the-mill person, whatever that means. It's not true. In fact, starting out knowing something they will have to learn has its strong points. You will already have the tools to make you more open to the many varieties of love. Love is not restricted to a set of rules. I will say this: The sooner you embrace the word *adopted,* the sooner you will find a defense that will help you grow into the loving man I know you can be.

Edited Out

I drove Mom home to Cove Street for our little ritual. The ocean was waiting behind Dad's picture window. I got two glasses of wine, and we sat down to Grammy Keaton's scrapbook, as usual. Mom was feeling proud of herself. She'd passed her periodic memory test with flying colors.

Dr. Cummings had presented a set of drawings with complex grids and intersecting lines, designed to confuse. Mother's assignment was to draw exactly what he'd drawn. The task was completed with few mistakes. First test down, two to go. The next section—always the hardest—required Dorothy to identify as many animals as she could in sixty seconds. She came up with cat, dog, elephant, lion, tiger, bear, reindeer, pig, and porcupine. Pretty darn good. When Cummings asked her to list as many words as possible that start with *F* in sixty seconds, Dorothy Deanne scored higher than expected.

Keep passing those tests, Mom. I hate them too. They continue to mount, not just for you but for Duke and Dex and me—well, everyone. It's rough. How about this one? Last week I plugged my ears in a bathroom stall at the Landmark Cinema when I heard someone say "Did you see Diane Keaton?" I couldn't help myself. I didn't want to hear what she might say. Some things never change. But forget about that; what I really hate are the mounting edits in our conversation. Neither one of us is passing that test. I know Duke's a nuisance you have a hard time tolerating. He's already caused you more confusion and more noise than Dexter ever did. I can't explain why he takes up so much space. I know you need my undivided attention. I just wish we could go back a couple of years. I'd love to get your take on him. For instance, I wish I could have talked to you about how I wound up with Duke's name.

First there was Parker, then Wade and Rover. I loved Clovis and Boeing, but Dorrie thought the reference to any kind of aircraft would bring us bad luck. I'm sure you would have approved of Cormac and Wimmer. But I bet names inspired from cities on the map, like Trancas and Butte, were pushing it, right? I considered Chester, Cleveland, Edison, and Ellis, then thought better. Too formal. I liked Hunter, but the connotations were creepy. I was mixed on Royce and Shane but loved Carter and Kendal. For a couple of days I was convinced his name had to be Walter, because of my long-standing crush on Walter Matthau. I wish we could have discussed the issue of Cash and Cameron and even Dewey. But Dewey was way too close to Dexie, who had some ideas of her own, including Tramp, and Mickey as in Mouse, but most of all Elmo. We would have had fun, Mom, but what's the point of rattling your brain when it might intrude on our glass of wine, and the big picture window, with the floating boats passing in honor of enjoying the calm before another storm, and the pride I know you feel for passing Dr. Cummings's memory test. Congratulations.

Message, 2001

"Diane, you're the hardest person to get ahold of. I hope you get this. I just want to congratulate you on being appointed to the Pasadena, no, no, no, to the, anyway, you're getting an award, or you're going to. Something's happening to you really big and good. I just want to congratulate you and root for you. Anyway, I'm home here. So maybe you could call me. Bye, Diane. Could you call me, Diane?"

Different Kinds of Bliss

I called Mom and told her I wasn't getting an award but I loved her congratulations. Yesterday I helped give her a sponge bath. Her breasts were like pendulums swinging back and forth. Had she wanted such big things so close to her heart? Every time I look at Duke or Dexter's flawless youth, I'm reminded of my own aging and how awful it is to witness what the human body comes to. Who am I if I don't recognize myself? Growing old, and I do mean growing, requires reinvention. In a way, growing old could be like joining Dexter on the Hurricane Harbor roller coaster—the ride of a lifetime, if I let myself go with it. I will say this: Growing old has made me appreciate things I wouldn't have expected to enjoy, like holding Mother's hand and trying to smooth out the folds of skin.

There's nothing to smooth out with Duke, whose crib sits in the middle of the closet next to my bedroom in the rented house on Elm Drive. Every morning he opens his eyes to an audience of hanging shirts and skirts. On the shelves above are dozens of hats. If he turns to the right, he sees the old Menendez Brothers' house out the window. It tells a dark story: Don't kill your parents. If he turns to the left, he sees me in the bedroom. It tells a happy story: Your mom loves you. Every morning I give him a kiss. Every morning he smiles, and I smile back. Simple, right? Wrong. With Duke there is no sixty-second time's-up within the free fall of his wonder. I grab him rough-house style and throw him on the bed. "You better not, Duke Radley Keaton. You better not."

He loves the veiled threat, almost as much as he loves going crazy mad screaming with laughter.

In between some serious skirmishes—like when he refuses to have his diaper changed, or when he starts crying because he's been put down or Dexter has stolen his waffle, or when he bangs his head on the sidewalk, or he doesn't get to pick worms out from under the concrete pavers in the front yard and I, the ogre, force him into his car seat, or I, the coldhearted, don't pay attention when attention must be paid—in between these scuffles, there are moments that feel like an eternity of bliss.

It was a different kind of bliss with Dexter at the swim meet, as I rubbed her back with sunscreen in the holding room at the indoor pool in Santa Clarita. Out of the blue, she suggested I take Lipitor. I looked over at the television screen mounted on a wall to see a fifty-something woman surfing a ten-footer in Hawaii as it cut to the word *Lipitor* in black. "Take it, Mom, you'll be stronger." "Thanks, Dex. Can I ask you something? When I'm eighty, will you still let me rub your back and kiss your sweet cheeks and hug you forever, even if you have a nice husband and two children of your own? Will you?" There was a long pause. "Mom, excuse me, but when you're gone, will I get all your money?"

I saw her dive into the water with dozens of other little sardines in bathing suits and caps. They swam in and out of the shadows cast from the skylight. Dexter caught the sun just as her arms stretched through the water of her designated lane. Heat 2, Lane 5. In that instant, she joined the other darling daughters racing upstream. So many girls swimming toward their destiny. For me, it was just one girl. Dexter.

Message, 2002

"Diane, this is your mom. I've been going through my checkbook, and I realized I made another mistake on the check I sent. I'm going to give up. I'm just going to give the whole thing up. I made it out for 200 million or something like that. I don't know—200 thousand? Would you check what you have, and call me back and tell me what my next move should be? I don't know why I can't get that into my head, but anyway, call me back, will you, as quick as you can, 'cause I'm sick of this. I'm going to close the books and never write another check. Okay, Diane . . . bye bye."

I'm Going to Miss You

I found cat feces in a plastic wineglass next to a pee-stained envelope of a long-forgotten bill addressed to Jack Hall. These are the days of derelict debris and a mounting stockpile of nonsense. Where's Irma, the new housekeeper? Anne Mayer, Mom's second daughter, as we call her, tells me Dorothy won't let Irma in. The rose-colored wall-to-wall carpet is filthy. I don't want Duke rolling around half naked on the surface of old cat poop. I knew I could lure Mom out of the house with the promise of a visit to her beloved Randy.

Everything was spotless when we returned. Mom shuffled into the kitchen, shaking her head as she held on to the walls for support. "Where am I?" She heaved a sigh and sat on the edge of the couch. "I don't know where I am. This isn't the place. Do I live here? I mean, I've been here before, but I don't live here now, right, Diane? That isn't my cat, even though it looks like a cat I would have. This is where we live? I can't put it together. Like right now, if you went off and left me here, I'd miss you, 'cause you wouldn't be there for me. Wait a minute. I think I've got it figured out. I'm in the living room, but I'm still confused. I'll tell you this: I'm going to miss you. What I want is to be somewhere comfortable with you. I kind of dread being here by myself. It disturbs me. I need company. I'm afraid, because I'm not real familiar with me. So, I'm here to stay? Is that it? What's later? I can't get a vision of how I'm going to make it work. I'm going to try to make the best of it though. It takes time to get things rolling again. Right? One more thing—could you tell me where my kids, Dorrie and Robin and Randy, are?"

Two Gifts and a Kiss, 2003

Nancy Meyers and I were having lunch. She'd become one of the few highly sought-out female directors after her debut with *Parent Trap,* starring Lindsay Lohan, followed by her $374 million blockbuster *What Women Want,* with Mel Gibson. In the interim, I'd made more money buying and selling houses than acting in a string of bombs, including *The Only Thrill, The Other Sister, Hanging Up* (which I also directed), and *Town & Country,* all critical and box-office failures. I was pretty much washed up as an actress and certainly as a fledgling director.

Over salad, Nancy told me she was writing a romantic comedy about a divorced playwright, Erica Barry, who falls in love with Harry Sanborn, a famous, womanizing owner of a record company. While Nancy filled me in on the details, I plotted career changes. Could I flip houses professionally? I needed an investor. I didn't want to keep restoring homes Dex and Duke and I lived in, only to sell them a year later. Was that good for the kids? When Nancy unequivocally said she wanted me to play Erica Barry and she was going to offer the part of Harry to Jack Nicholson, I snapped out of it. "Wait a minute. Jack Nicholson? I'm sorry, but Jack Nicholson is not going to play my boyfriend in a chick flick. That's not his thing. Nancy, you're brilliant, and I'm totally thrilled you want me, but there's no way he's going to accept your offer, which is just another way of saying you'll never get the financing either. So I wouldn't bother getting your hopes up. Don't even try." I left knowing her untitled film project would never see the light of day. And, frankly, I wished she'd never told me. I didn't want to hold on to a pipe dream. A year and a half later, Jack and I started shooting *Something's Gotta Give* on the Sony lot.

As I left the Hôtel Plaza Athénée in Paris for the last night of principal photography on *Something's Gotta Give,* I was greeted by a phalanx of paparazzi hoping for Cameron Diaz, who was at the hotel, or Jack, only to find themselves in front of a solitary Diane Keaton—or was it Diane Lane, as my invitation to the Valentino Fall Collection was addressed. It had been a long shoot, six months to be exact. After our last shot, Jack hugged me goodbye, saying something about a little piece. I hugged him back and we went our separate ways. Two years later, a check with a lot of zeroes arrived in the mail for my back-end percentage on *Something's Gotta Give*. I didn't have a back-end deal. There must have been some mistake. I called my business manager, who told me it was from Jack Nicholson. Jack? That's when I remembered him saying something about a little piece when we hugged goodbye. Oh, my God. He meant he was going to give me a piece of his own percentage.

There were so many contradictions and inconsistencies with Jack. So many surprises. One day we were shooting on the set of Erica's beach house. The script described the scene as: "Erica and Harry, wet from the rain, quickly shut all the doors and windows. Lightning crackles across the sky and the lights in the house go out. A match is struck and a candle is lit. Then another one, and another one. Erica turns and finds Harry just looking at her. Before either of them has time to think, they kiss." For me, Diane, not Erica, the kiss was a reigniting reminder of something lost suddenly found. "I'm sorry," Erica says. "For what?" Harry says. "I just kissed you," Erica says. "No, honey, I kissed you," Harry says. Then, as scripted, Erica kisses Harry. Instantly I, Diane, forgot my next line. "Damn it, I'm sorry. What do I say?" The script supervisor whispered, " 'I know that one was me.' " In other words, I, Diane, or rather I, Erica Barry, took the lead and kissed Harry first. We tried the take one more time. As soon as I kissed Jack—or, rather, Harry—I forgot the line again. "I'm sorry. I don't know what's going on here. What's the line one more time?" From her director's chair in Video Village Nancy shouted, "Diane, it's 'I know that one was me.'" "Right. Oh, right, right, of course. I'm sorry, Nancy. Let me try it again." This went on for another ten minutes. I honestly didn't know what I was doing. The only thing I remembered was not to forget to kiss Jack. Kissing him within the safety of a story that wasn't mine, even though it felt like it was, was exhilarating. I forgot I was in a movie. Nancy's story was merging into my story—Diane's story of a kiss with Jack, aka Harry. And the great thing was, Harry aka Jack had to love it just as much as I, Diane, aka Erica, had to love it. I don't know what Jack, not Harry, felt. I just know everything that came out of his mouth gave me the rush of a "first-time love" over and over. It wasn't the script. It was Jack. And Jack can't be explained.

So that's what *Something's Gotta Give* gave me: Nancy's godsend, Jack's kiss, and a piece of the back end. *Something's Gotta Give* will always be my favorite movie, not only because it was so unexpected at age fifty-seven, but also because it gave me the wonderful feeling of being in the presence of a couple of extraordinary people who delivered two gifts and a kiss.

A Different Message, 2005

The new nurse left a message before she quit. "Your mother appears to have a lot of hallucinations. When she took the lorazepam, she screamed and started staggering. Her arms shook too. If she wanted something, she let out a scream. She held on to the pull bar and wouldn't let go. She kept screaming 'No' over and over and said the wall was moving. She saw people in the room. I don't think this medication is working."

Maybe that's the reason Mom was reeling around half mad yesterday. She didn't care if Dad's ashes were scattered on the hill in Tubac or not, she was going to sell the house, and she was going to cut down the star pine they'd planted on the terrace too. "Mom, sit down. Let's talk about it. Eat." But, no, she was up to get something she'd forgotten, saying, "What is that thing you cook with? What is it? Who's that boy? Shut up, little boy." Duke started to cry. I told him not to worry, I'd take him for a walk to Big Corona. Dexter whispered, "Mama, ask Gramma if I can have a Coke." Mom spun around. "What is she doing? Why is she telling you secrets in front of me?" "She wants a Coke, Mom." "Well, why doesn't she ask me? Speak up, young lady, you're in my house." "She knows, Mom. I think she's feeling a little shy." "Well, if she doesn't want to talk to me, she shouldn't come over. I can tell she doesn't even like me. Do you, little girl? Do you? What's your problem anyway?" Dexter froze. Duke tugged at me. "Mama. Come." We left.

It was hard to watch Mother struggle with the constant agitation she couldn't comprehend. The slow picking away plopped her smack dab into the late middle stages of Alzheimer's, maybe even early late. I don't know, and I don't want to. When Duke, Dexter, and I said goodbye after our walk to Big Corona, Mother had forgotten we'd left, or even that we'd been there, for that matter. She was sitting in the living room, staring into space. When I kissed her, she wanted to know what group I was with.

Chubby Cheeks, 2006

What group are you with, Duke? I know the answer: You're with the group called inception. You're with the beginning. I kiss you good morning. You rub my cheek and say, "It's what your cheek wants." "Really, how about a kiss for Mom?" "No. You get what you get, and you don't get more, cheek stealer." "That's not the way to talk to your mother, Mr. Man. And what's with the cheeks? Now, c'mon, let's get going and have some breakfast." I frown big-time. You laugh as you run into the kitchen and open the Traulsen freezer, grab two SpongeBob Popsicles, and yell, "Save it for the movies, Mom." "Put them back, Duke Radley, and guess what, breakfast is for healthy food, not Popsicles or frozen mini mint pancakes. How about some oatmeal?" "Mom, you know what's bad about your name? Die. Die. Die. Mom, when you die and I die, will we still be able to think?" "I hope so, Duke. Please don't climb on the countertop."

Dexter, not a morning person, appears grim-faced as she heads for the Life cereal. You say you'll eat the oatmeal but only if you can add a serving of Cinnamon Crunch and two sugar cubes. "Okay, okay," I say, and turn on CNN, while pouring soy milk into a bowl, which I put in the microwave. I watch you press CLEAR, then 2, then 1, then START, then STOP, and then repeat the whole process all over again.

"Twenty-one seconds, right, Mom?" "Twenty-one, not forty-two, Duke." Finally you sit down, take a bite, then tell me how fat your tummy is. "Mom." "What?" "Why does it have to end with your cheeks?"

The kitchen door swings open. Lindsay Dwelley walks in, already exhausted. You whisper, "I wish Lindsay was separated from Lindsay." Dexter sticks her foot out. You trip. "Dexter, I saw that. That's a time-out." Dexter screams, "Duke's an idiot," and runs off. "Mom, does Dexter creep you out, or is it just me?" "Duke. That's enough smart talk." "But, Mom, you're so complicated. You've got to snap out of it." "Duke. Dang it, Christ. That's enough! Time-out for you too, buddy." "Mom, I won't say 'Dang it, Christ,' if you don't. I won't say 'stupid jerk' if you don't. I won't say 'fuuuuuuu' "—you stop yourself—"if you don't. Got it, Mama Cheeks? Fair enough?" "Duke, I'm not going to say it one more time—GO UPSTAIRS." You head out, but not before grabbing as many action figures as your hands can hold. "I'm sorry, Mom, but honestly, I mean, what does a man have to do to get help with his luggage?" "UPSTAIRS." "I'm sorry, Mom. I'm sorry. When you die I'll be so sad, but at least I'll be able to touch your cheeks without asking."

Frank Mancuso Jr. and Mount Rushmore

When did Suzy Dionicio, Mom's new caregiver, start dripping food into the right side of Mom's mouth three times a day every day? Breakfast takes an hour and a half. Lunch and dinner two. Suzy is patient, knowing Mom has a hard time remembering to swallow. After the meds have been mashed into a thickened tea for Mom to sip, Suzy turns on the new flat-screen TV to PBS so Mom can look at the primary colors on *Sesame Street*. After she pulls all 130 pounds of Dorothy Deanne's five-feet-seven-inch frame onto the Hoyer lift, she watches her mamacita rise like a phoenix. It's as if a giant baby with a long white pigtail is gliding across the room in a computer-driven stork. Suzy's navigational skills plop Dorothy into the wheelchair, where her head lands with a thud on her chest. How will Mom see all the colors if her view is limited to the discounted tile floor she and Dad fought over?

In between the joy of the kids and the heartbreak of Mom's decline, there was the day I couldn't remember the name of Mount Rushmore. A few weeks before, Frank Mancuso Jr.'s name went missing too. On the one hand, who cares? Is Frank Mancuso storage-worthy? When you consider all the things that need to be addressed, why flog myself for forgetting someone I don't really know or care about?

When does "Where did I put my keys?" become a diagnosis? Will I be joining Mom in the fog of forgetting? Will our family's genetic profile snatch my memory away too? Do I have it already? I've stopped telling people my mother has Alzheimer's disease. It turns an otherwise simple encounter into the beginning of what feels like, that's right, a test. Will I pass?

Does the effect of accumulated self-doubt create a form of depression that leads to Alzheimer's disease? I know I keep asking, but does it? That's the only answer I can come up with. I know I'm grabbing at straws, but really!!! I know,

I know, learn to live with the questions. But, seriously, does one's psychological profile play a part? And if it does, would this knowledge have changed things for Mom? God knows taking vitamin E and ginkgo and Aricept and two glasses of wine a day didn't do one bit of good. Just as advanced language skills, education, and even genius didn't stop Ralph Waldo Emerson, Iris Murdoch, E. B. White, or Somerset Maugham from the "insidious onset." Consider this: Speaking is present tense. Writing exists in thought. They wrote. Adding voice to ideas gives words vitality. Of course, speaking is not a cure for Alzheimer's, but it is a vital component in the battle against depression and anxiety, both of which dogged Mother. I've always had trouble putting words together. In a way, I became famous for being an inarticulate woman. The disparity between Mom and me is that I got my feelings out. I memorized other people's words and made them feel like my own. Writing is abstract. I'm sure I'm wrong, but to think of my mother, a person who loved words, got A's, went back to college in her forties, and came home with a diploma, as another victim of Alzheimer's disease without a clear-cut reason is something I can't accept.

I hate the fact that Mom's middle years under the auspices of Alzheimer's have ended. What does she get in return? The famous blank stare, that's what she gets; another face of forgetting. Give me back the years of agitation, anything over the soothing shield of apathy and silence. Fuck it. What's the point of my questions and potential answers to something that can't be explained? It's a fruitless enterprise. All of it. I just want Mom's brain back.

Get this: As Duke and I were waiting in line at Jamba

Juice this afternoon, my cellphone rang. It was Stephanie, the captain of Team Keaton. Did I remember the conference call with Michael Gendler? I was about to say yes, but Frank Mancuso Jr.'s name popped up as Duke dropped his aloha pineapple vanilla smoothie all over the floor. Mount Rushmore and Frank Mancuso Jr. came rushing back. They'd been saved from obscurity, but only after I let them go.

14
THEN AGAIN

Family

I was on my cellphone in the car, going over the endless to-do list with Stephanie. "Can you believe the alarm went off at four A.M. yet again? That's three times in two weeks. What's going on? All I can say is, thank God the kids slept through it. Anyway, please get the alarm guy to come over today and fix the damn thing. Okay? Oh, and I've got to reschedule dinner with Sarah Paulsen; plus, return the call to John Fierson. Do you have his number? Dang it. Hold on for a sec? Someone's calling. Shoot, I've got a zillion things to go over with you. Don't go away. Never mind. I'll call you right back."

It was Anne Mayer. She was saying something about Mom having bronchitis. She was aspirating. "Anyway, they admitted her into Hoag Hospital. But Dr. Berman thinks she'll be home by tomorrow." As I turned the car around and headed for Hoag, I forgot about the to-do list.

When I found Mom, she was plugged into an IV. Some sort of machine had been placed over her nose and mouth to help loosen the phlegm. The X-rays revealed evidence of a recent, undetected stroke. There was no indication of pneumonia, but Mom couldn't swallow. Without taking extraordinary measures, there was nothing more Hoag could do. Mother would be released. That meant hospice, and hospice meant morphine.

I went home, packed a bag, and headed to Cove, where I found everything once again transformed. The word *stuff* came to mind. Stuff and junk—not the kind you collect but the kind you throw away. Old medicine bottles. Broken plates. Too many Kleenex boxes on the bed stand. Caregivers' logs. Too many ugly balloons and awful floral arrangements. This wasn't a celebration. Mom's beloved home was stuffed with the effects of illness. If she were cognizant, she wouldn't have allowed Suzy D to throw a sheet over the picture window, nor would the ancient videos of my films be collecting dust in the cabinets Dorothy so carefully designed. But it was the sight of Mom's mottled hands holding a cute little stuffed bunny next to her chest that just about did me in. "Isn't it pretty, Diane! If you pull the cord it plays 'Mockingbird.' "

Robin had flown in from Atlanta with Riley. Randy walked around with a Rolling Rock beer as he smiled at Claudia, his friend. Anne Mayer, Suzy D, and Irma were also in attendance. Out of the corner of my eye, I saw Charlotte, the hospice nurse, try to drip morphine under Mom's tongue.

Morphine and Ativan every two hours. Suzy tried to help widen Dorothy's clenched jaw. "Open your mouth, Mamacita. We love our Mamacita, don't we, Dorrie?" Dorrie nodded.

Stephanie called. The unanswered to-do list was waiting. Mom didn't have Internet access. Just as well. In her workroom, surrounded by stacks of carousels filled with slides from the sixties of Randy, Robin, Dorrie, and me catching waves at San Onofre, I told Stephanie I was going to take a break.

Dad would have loved Google and Twitter and Facebook and the BlackBerry. He would have been taken by the immediate everything, the instant history, the access to anywhere across all continents. Still, the dilemma is the same as it always was: What to do? How do we focus on some aspect of information that will help forge a path to an emotionally fulfilling life? Dorothy knew it was a matter of picking and choosing. She never quite figured out a way to find an audience for the missing part, the part that made her feel she was enough. She lost something on the way. Mom's strength as a writer came out of assemblage. She understood the transitory nature and impact of information. In one ear, out the other. At heart, she was a modernist without the craft to gather her insights into a cohesive message. From Mom's brain to the world. From the outer reaches of her mind's impulses to her silent audience. The incoming messages. The outgoing summing up of a life.

She knew one thing: It all boils down to family. One day you end up having spent your life with a handful of people. I did. I have a family—two, really. Well, three if you think about it. There are my siblings, and there are my children, but I also have an extended family. The people who stayed. The people who became more than friends; the people who open the door when I knock. That's what it all boils down to. The people who have to open the door, not because they always want to but because they do.

A Balloon

Four days have passed since our band of caretakers decided to hang in for the duration. Sometimes we sleep on the couch downstairs or in the storage room with Mom's old file cabinets. Sometimes we share our parents' king-size bed. Sometimes Suzy D spends the night, other times Anne and Irma too. The hospice nurses come and go, carrying little vials of morphine in their handbags. Yesterday the kids came for a visit. Robin and I were watching them play at the shoreline when we heard Anne screaming. Robin grabbed my hand. We rushed past Don Callender, heir to Marie Callender pies, propped in a wheelchair. He made a gesture not quite capable of being called a wave. Running past, I thought of all those frozen pies sold to all those millions of American consumers. Money couldn't help him now. He tried to speak. What was he saying? Robin gripped me. "Diane, come on. Hurry."

Inside, Dorrie, Suzy, Irma, Anne, and Riley were gathered around the hospital bed. Mom's breathing was irregular. Charlotte, the nurse, checked her stopwatch at every inhalation. Mom would take a breath, hold it for thirty-five seconds before exhaling to take another, hold it for thirty seconds, then take another for fifty. Having had asthma, I knew how hard it was to work for so little air. Inhale, hold for thirty. Exhale. Inhale, hold for forty. Exhale. Inhale, hold for thirty-eight. We looked for a pattern. We waited. When she took a breath and held it for sixty-five seconds, Dorrie started to cry. Robin pressed her face against Mother's cheek. Duke, with a towel around his shoulders, came running in. "Mommy, don't cry. Don't cry, Mommy." I hugged him tight and kissed his seven-and-a-half-year-old body. Was this the end? Duke untied a helium balloon at the end of the bed and pushed its words, GET WELL, close to Mom's face. "Get well, Grammy. See, it says 'Get well.'" Mom, as if hearing his plea, didn't die. But it made me think of the others who already had.

Some Deaths

First Mike

Mike Carr, my cousin, died in 1962. He was fourteen. Mom, Dad, Randy, Robin, Dorrie, and I piled out of our Buick station wagon and entered the mid-century A-frame church still standing on the outskirts of Garden Grove, California. We sat in a pew close to Auntie Martha. She wasn't crying, but her face looked unfamiliar. It was as if she'd been dealt a blow too hard to assimilate. Martha Carr was never the same, not ever, ever, ever. Something was broken that could never be repaired. The minister's message was filled with Bible quotes chosen for funerals. There was no mention of the allegations that Mike accidentally shot himself with a rifle during an acid trip in Seattle.

Then Eddie

Aunt Sadie's husband, Eddie, went next. Grammy Hall hated Eddie. After thirty years, she finally convinced Sadie to kick him out of the duplex. According to Mary, "men don't count for much." Eddie and George were weak; why else would they cling to women with means like her? When Eddie died in his cabin up in June Lake, there were no hard feelings between him and Sadie; he left all of his paint-by-number landscapes to her and their son, Cousin Charlie.

Then George

One thing about George, Grammy's boarder: He never failed to give us kids the best birthday cards. They always pictured different kinds of trees filled with a dollar's worth of dimes in the branches. We called them the money-tree cards.

George was a painter, a housepainter. He was also a member of the painters' union. Every Christmas, the union threw a big bash with a giant Christmas tree and tons of presents for all the children. An announcer hosted my favorite part, the talent show. He carried a big silver microphone with a long cord and asked if anyone wanted to get up and sing. I never had the nerve, but I wanted to. I really wanted to. I used to wish Daddy had joined the union. I wanted him to dance and do funny voices like George. George did card tricks too.

Grammy didn't say much when George got skinny. The morning he keeled over and died, Grammy didn't cry. "He never gave me a dime. Not one dime." That's all she said. I thought of the money-tree cards. I wished I hadn't spent all those dimes. I would have given them to Grammy so she wouldn't be so angry about George. After all, he died. I was sure George meant for her to have as many dimes as she wanted. And even if he didn't, he always tried to pay his rent on time. Grammy's response was hard for me to decipher. Why wasn't she sad? It wasn't nice. What it was was cold and unattended, like her duplex on Range View Avenue.

Then Sadie

"Ninety-three years is no small eggs, but what does it matter now that Sadie's gone?" Grammy Hall paused. "There ain't much left in a way. I'll tell you one thing. There's no sense in worrying about dying. A lot of people ain't got very good minds on the subject. I say don't be overactive in thinking, Diane, because you can think so much your mind goes hay-wire. I can't get Sadie's pacemaker out of my mind. It wasn't pulling its weight. She had a little button for the damn thing. She was always fiddling with that button, you know. Rolling it around and around. Then she started acting stupid for about a week. I never thought much about it. I went to the store, and when I came back she was dead. She had on a pink dress. I think she put on that dress 'cause she knew her time was up. I hate to say it, but the truth is, Sadie got taken up in the whodunit of an all too predictable death."

Even Dr. Landau Too

Dr. Landau was diagnosed with Alzheimer's disease. She told me she was retiring but she would still like to see me in her apartment at 96th Street and Madison. On our last visit, she was telling me the story of how she and her husband, Marvin, had escaped Poland on the eve of Hitler's invasion, when out of the blue she began speaking in a language I couldn't identify. I pretended to understand what she was saying by nodding my head and smiling in what I thought was a soothing manner. Even with Alzheimer's, Dr. Landau didn't suffer fools. She glared at me as if I was deliberately putting her on. She wasn't wrong, but what the heck was she saying? No matter how much I tried to placate her, she got more unnerved, so much so that she started to point her finger at me and scream as if I'd betrayed her. A nurse appeared and took her away. Dr. Landau, like Mary Hall, did not look back. We didn't say goodbye, and I never saw her again.

In better days, Dr. Landau explained there was no such thing as fair. I didn't agree. Life had to have its reasons. It couldn't be a lawless jumble of contradictions. As I watched her shuffle out of her living room, holding on to her caregiver's arm amid the orange and black furniture she'd spent years collecting, I couldn't believe the woman who'd spent her entire adult life helping people battle the insistent demons playing havoc with their minds had been struck down by Alzheimer's. It would take twenty years before Mother would be joining her in the fluster and distress of a shrinking brain. Felicia Lydia Landau was right; life is not fair.

One Phone Call, Two Messages, September 8, 2008

On the seventh day of our encampment on Cove Street, I went to pick up some lunch from Baja Fresh while Suzy sprayed Mother's hair with dry shampoo and freshened her braid. The signs couldn't be clearer. Low blood pressure. Low pulse rate. A waxy surface spreading across her face. Poor circulation. Dehydration. Every hour, on the hour, as if there was some reasonable order to the process, Dorothy's gurgling sound got louder.

When I got back, there was a message from the kids. "Hi, Mom, it's Dexter. Today was such a great day at the beach. I caught a six-foot wave with a four-and-a-half-foot drop. Oh, my God. Everyone was like, 'Dude, that was sick.' It was, like, sooo awesome. The boogie-boarding waves were soooo good. Whoo-hoo. I'm a beast in the water. I don't think I'll ever stop being a water bug. Tomorrow should be the same. Please, oh, please, let there be big waves. Here's Duke." "Mom, come home. Where are you? I want to sleep with you tonight. Can we *all* sleep together? I get to sleep in the middle. Mama, I wanted to say something. I'm having the Irish oatmeal. And, Mama, I wanted to say that when you get home I want to play with you for a little. And, Mom, there's something else I wanted to say—Dexter is evil. Bye."

We ate tacos around the dining room table. Everyone looked worse for the wear. Robin went to drop Riley off at the airport. Dorrie left to get more supplies. The caregivers took a break. It was Mom and me alone together for the last time. I looked at her face, not her ice-cold ankles, or her yellow feet. Nature had been so damn inconsistent. How ironic that Mom's handsome face made it all but impossible for people to trace the fragile soul hiding behind such stature. I leaned in close. Safe within the perimeter of Mother's pale aspect, I wondered what she'd seen before her eyes shut. Had the landscape of bobbing, once-loved faces been an intrusion, all those perplexed nodding heads? Mom, what do you hear in the land of no words? The dishes being washed? The ocean pounding against the seawall? Does the chorus of voices whispering "Mamacita" and "Morning, Mom" and "Dear, dear Dorothy" and "Mrs. Hall" mean anything at all?

Alone together, I hope you can identify our voices. Or are we another refrain you can't make out? If sound is the last thing to go, I hope our chorus soothes you. It's our lullaby of heartache. Can you hear us cooing? Does it reverberate? It's our song of loving you from the other side of your white sheet.

I guess it's safe to assume your eyes won't be opening anytime soon, will they, Mom? I see you're still clenching your jaw. No one's messed with that mouth of yours since the day you bit Suzy D's finger. "Dorothy's Last Stand," that's what Dorrie called it. I wish you didn't have to grip so hard. I know you're trying to hold on to what little is left. I would too. I'm sorry there's only one door left for you to open.

Everything seems arbitrary and haphazard and distorted

and out of whack. Remember Grammy Hall harping about "health is wealth"? Only now do I know what she meant. Duke and Dexter are covered by a host of physicians. There's Dr. Sherwood, Dexter's orthodontist, and Christie Kidd for her skin care. There's Dr. Peter Waldstein, Duke's pediatrician, and Dr. Randy Schnitman for his many ear infections. As for me, the doctor list gets longer and longer. There's my dentist, Dr. James Robbins, who recently made me a bite plate; yes, I grind my teeth. There's his wife, Rose, the dental hygienist; and Dr. Keith Agre, my internist. Dr. Silverman gives me the yearly eye examination. There's ninety-six-year-old Dr. Leo Rangell, my irreplaceable psychoanalyst. And I can't leave out Dr. Bilchick, for my sprouting garden of skin cancers.

Remember my first squamous cell at twenty-one, followed by a series of basal cell carcinomas in my thirties? Warren used to bug me all the time about sitting in the sun. Why didn't I listen? This year, more than forty years later, that mean-spirited invasive squamous cell revisited the left side of my face. I drove to Cedars-Sinai, put on a shower cap, and lay down on the gurney. As the anesthesiologist injected me, I began to drift through a kind of flip book of images. I saw you, just like me, lying on a gurney, only you weren't alive. I saw Dad on a gurney too. I saw the extra-long needle putting Red-dog to sleep. Should I have given him more treats? I saw my friend Robert Shapizon sitting under his Andy Warhol with the giant dollar sign, discussing the emotional effects of inoperable lung cancer. Why hadn't I spent more time with him? I saw Larry Sultan holding the cover of his book *Evidence* as everything started to go black. That's when I swear I heard Larry's voice say he wanted to live three more weeks, just three more weeks. It wasn't like he was asking for much. . . . When I woke up, I had a four-inch scar running down my face. Life is starting to chip away at me too, Mom. This living stuff is a lot. Too much, and not enough. Half empty, and half full.

The Day Before

Suzy called from downstairs. She was looking for a pair of tweezers. I went into Mom's workroom. It's funny how you overlook the obvious. Along with THINK, Scotch-taped to the wall was a quote I'd never seen. "Memories are simply moments that refuse to be ordinary." I hope Mom has kept a few tucked away in some retrievable part of her mind. Hunting around, I came across a few random pages Mom wrote after Dad died.

Cyrus, the cat, was mercifully and painlessly put to sleep this morning. This is a statement of sorrow at losing my beautiful Abyssinian cat, a real cat who understood his position in life and until his death did his job magnificently. I already miss him.

I don't know why the verse from Ecclesiastes, Chapter 3, came to me as I sat in a hot bath trying to get over the fact that Cyrus is no longer alive, but it did. I got out of the tub, picked up my mother's old Bible, and found it. "To everything there is a season, and a time to every purpose under Heaven. A time to be born, and a time to die; a time

to weep and a time to laugh; a time to mourn, a time to
dance. A time to get and a time to lose."

I find peace in these words, probably because death is a
mystery and at times a torturous burden to live with. It's so
hard to understand the complexities of our human exis-
tence. Why were we created with emotions of love only to
be left with such emptiness when those we have felt love for
are taken out of our lives? I will never know the answer
until I die and join those who have gone before me: Jack,
Mother, Mary, Sadie, Cyrus the cat, and quite probably I,
next.

The Long Haul

After eleven days, Suzy D's incessant "Praise the Lord, I pray
for our Mamacita morning, noon, and night, God bless Dorothy" rant was driving me nuts, so nuts that I put my finger
in Mother's mouth, hoping she'd bite me, just to shake things
up, but Mom's fight-back spirit was gone. I was free to feel
the jagged edges of her teeth. She was flunking her last test,
or maybe she passed it and was ready to let go in order to
join Jack.

Dorrie and I pushed her hospital bed in front of the picture window, where we tore off the hanging sheet. Enough
with the darkness. What exactly had we been protecting
Mother from? Certainly not the sun. With Mom only three
feet away from Dad's picture window, Dorrie and I stood
looking at our still life. That's what she'd become—a still

life, a painting, an object. What did any of our gestures matter? Picture window or not, prolonging Mother's life felt like cruelty, even a form of subdued torture.

We washed and bathed her. We held her hand as she was turned from one side to another every hour on the hour. We swabbed her mouth with a wet sponge. The hospice nurses administered morphine. Dr. Berman consoled us much in the same manner Dad's doctor at UCLA had done. It was the quality of life. The quality of life? As far as I could see, there was no quality left for Mom. She couldn't swallow. She couldn't speak. She couldn't see. The only part of her body that moved was her left hand, and its only function had been reduced to clutching the railing of the hospital bed. Now, with our mother's face directed toward the warmth of the sun, she no longer clutched the railing either.

September 18, 2008

Sitting at the edge of the bed, I monitored Dorothy's condition while Suzy D went upstairs. She was holding steady at sixteen breaths per minute. I didn't see it coming. There was no sign. Only when the purple in her hands began to fade did I understand Mother had passed away without so much as a single involuntary sound.

We dressed her in brown wool pants, with a white shirt and an old black sweater embroidered with a green cactus. Her braid was perfectly straight, like her patrician nose. All dressed up in her desert go-to-dinner outfit, with lipstick highlighting her no-longer-blue lips. Robin, Dorrie, and I drank red wine behind the picture window. We waited for the man from the Neptune Society to push her through the living room, past the two club chairs we bought at Pottery Barn, just like Dad before her.

I went home the next morning and told Duke and Dexter that "Grammy's heart slowed down, and she stopped breathing. She had a good ending." "Grammy had a good ending?" "Yes, Dex." "She didn't deserve to die," Duke said. I told him once again how her heart slowed down. But this time I added the miracles. I talked about the day her fingertips started to turn crimson, and how as time passed the color slowly began to crawl up her arms and legs, and how her body began to look like a beautiful plum. That was the first miracle. Then I told them how things changed on the night of Grammy's death. Her lips turned an indigo blue like the ocean at sunset. I told them I didn't know the exact moment Grammy passed away, because I was distracted by the sudden sound of flapping wings. I looked outside and there in the dark was a swarm of seagulls standing on the deck, as if they were trying to say goodbye to the nice lady who used to throw bread crumbs on the seawall's deck. When I turned back and saw Grammy's arms, then hands, and even her ocean-blue lips return to normal, I knew I was in the presence of a miracle. But the biggest miracle came when I looked into her eyes: The same beautiful brown eyes that had been closed for seven long days and seven long nights were open. Wide open. I asked Dexter and Duke if they thought their grandmother might have been seeing something she'd never seen before. They both agreed she must have been looking into something on the other side of new.

I didn't tell them Mother's death was as inexplicable as the life she lived right down to her last undetermined breath. I didn't tell them how the door stood open for twelve days. I didn't tell them Mom stepped in and closed it behind her without so much as a murmur.

Little Goodbyes

I've been opening and closing doors all my life. But the door marked LETTING GO has remained shut. Writing the story of Mom's story was not intended to underscore loss over other aspects. I didn't plan on an elegy. Still, Dad's five-month sprint to goodbye, followed by Mom's protracted journey to farewell, had a cumulative effect.

My belated hello to a baby girl and boy created different kinds of endings. I call them the Little Goodbyes, like the day Dexter stopped getting into bed with me at three A.M., and the day *Stellaluna* was put on the bookshelf for good. There was the day Dexter caught seven butterflies with her bare hands. Goodbye, butterflies. There was the last time she said, "Good night, Dorrie, and Ray [Dorrie's dog], and Mojo [her other dog], and Shatah [her ugly dog]. Good night to Steve Shadley Designs, and Uncle Bill [Robinson], and Grammy, and Lindsay, and Uncle Johnny Gale, and TaTa, and Sandra, especially Sandra." There was the day I brought a brand-new Duke Radley home from New York City. That was the day Dexter said goodbye to being an only child. There was the day Duke said his first word. "Moon." There was the day he was twelve months old. I want back the last day Dexter and I sneaked into the former Jimmy Stewart house, under construction on Roxbury, and the day Duke and I were in the backyard looking at the sky when he said, "We will keep lying down on the grass in order to look at the sky forever, right, Mom?" "Sure, Duke, of course, always." I can't remember the day Dexter stopped saying "Member." "Member how Josie threw up in the car?" "Member the bird's nest we found?" No more "member"s, Dexie. There was the afternoon she didn't want to dive for plastic elephants at the bottom of the pool. Goodbye, elephants, and crocodiles too. There was the day Duke stopped watching *Kipper* and *Thomas the Tank Engine* videos, and the day he forgot to beg me to play "Come into my house." Goodbye, little cardboard house. There was the last day we sang "Gillis Mountain" as we tooled along in my big black Defender. That was the day I cranked the volume as high as it would go, so we could scream out the words "I took a trip up Gillis Mountain on a sunny summer day." Goodbye, Gillis Mountain. Goodbye. You'd think the accumulation of so many little goodbyes would have prepared me for the bigger ones, but they didn't.

It all comes back to the same old thing, Mom. I wish we could talk. I wish I could hear what you might want to tell me from the other side of nowhere. Your last lesson, the one I can't bear to acknowledge and refuse to identify, is beginning to take hold. I think I know what you want to say from THEN. That's where you are, isn't it? You're in THEN. From there I bet you want to tell me to lift my hands off the handlebars of the bike and let go. You want to say, "Diane, don't cover your ears; listen. Don't close your eyes; look. Don't shut your mouth; open it wide and speak." You want to say, "Dear Diane, my firstborn, take a deep breath, be brave, and let go. Release your hands from their grip on the bike, lift them up and fly."

I'm trying, Mom, but it goes against every instinct I possess. I promise you one thing though. I promise to unleash Duke and Dexter from the stranglehold of my need before it's too late. I promise to give them their freedom no matter how much I want them to hang on. I promise to let go of you too, the you I created for the benefit of me. I only wish that once, just once, I had the courage to say what I felt as I averted my eyes and waved goodbye. You see, Mom, it was always you. It was you for as long as long is.

Where Are They Now?

Yesterday, Nick Reid photographed Mom's journal from 1968 on a tabletop he devised in Duke and Dexter's playroom. The cover of the black-ringed binder is a collage filled with photographs of Randy, Robin, Dorrie, and me in gangster getups, à la Bonnie and Clyde. "It's a Great Year So Far" is pasted at the bottom left-hand corner. "Cut Loose" is at the top right. On the title page inside are the words WHERE ARE THEY NOW?

Here's where we are, Mom. Robin is sixty. Can you believe she's been married to Rickey Bevington for twenty-seven years? Impossible, right? They still live on their forty-seven-acre farm in Sharpsburg, Georgia. Her baby, Jack, is going to college, and twenty-one-year-old Riley has a new baby named Dylan. Robin continues to carry on your penchant for collecting stray dogs and cats. She has thirteen.

Dorrie wakes up to a perfect view of the San Gabriel mountain range, like you used to when you were a girl. She loves her tree house high on top of a hill in Silver Lake. As the CEO of Monterey Garage Designs, she remains a premier dealer as well as collector of the American West, specializing in Monterey furniture. She loves to drive to the Tubac, Arizona, home with her dogs Cisco and Milo. You would be proud of her, Mom.

Randy still has that rusty Toyota van Dad gave him. It's been sitting in his carport for fifteen years. Typical, right? His new apartment in Belmont Village is jammed with what must be thousands of collages, and books, and torn-out magazines and weird frames, and paintbrushes and glue, and, well, ephemera everywhere. He still keeps his poems in the oven. I finally got him on the phone the other day. You know what he said? He said he's never been happier. How about that, Mom?

I'm okay, but it's Christmas, and your ashes are in the back of my Tahoe Hybrid. We're driving you to Tubac, where Robin, Dorrie, and I will spread your remains next to Dad's. I found an old tin cross at Architectural Salvage in Minneapolis last fall. We painted your name across the surface. "Dorothy Deanne Keaton Hall. Beloved Mother to daughter Dorrie, daughter Diane, son Randy, daughter Robin." You'll be overlooking the Santa Rita mountain range up in the high desert along with Dad and his traveling companion.

I'm on the road with Duke, my very own Junior Jim Carrey, and Dexter, my Teen Queen. Every day I check out their faces, looking for signs of change. I look at their perfect noses, their radiant smiles, their thick hair. I scan Dexter's wide-set eyes and Duke's gorgeous cleft chin. Do they have to grow up? Why am I so fortunate? How did these two choices thrust me out of a life of isolation into a kind of family-of-man scenario, complete with an extended family, new friends, and much needed ordinary activities? How is it possible I became one of those swim-meet moms, driving Duke to Santa Clarita at seven A.M., only to find myself standing in the rain watching Dexter swim the 400 free at five P.M.? Wish you could have been there. Wish you could have seen Duke and Dexter stretch their perfect bodies and dive into that cold water. Wish you could have come to Hawaii too. That would have been fun. You could have ordered pineapple snow cones under the waterfall. You could have watched them fly down the water slide, laughing all the way. You could have joined us on the boat ride from hell with the Iraqi war-vet tour guides tossing us up and down at sixty miles an hour in ten-foot swells.

One more thing, Mom. How does it all so soon become then? I guess there's a consolation. It's weird, but I think you'll understand. As I've written our memoir—your words with my words—sometimes I feel like it's Again without the Then. Do you understand what I'm saying? Can you hear me? I'm saying I'm with you again. THEN. AGAIN. Then again, Mom. Then again.

IN MEMORY OF

DR. LEO RANGELL. ROBERT SHAPAZIAN. MICHAEL BALOG. LARRY SULTAN. MAURY CHAYKIN. MARTHA CARR. MIKE CARR. RED. ALAN BUCHSBAUM. MAHALA HOIEN. NANCY SHORT. DAVID MCCLOUD. GEORGE. AND EDDIE. ROY KEATON. FRANK ZIMMERMAN. DR. FELICIA LANDAU. SANDY MEISNER. AND SADIE. DOMINO. JOSIE. WHITEY. WALTER MATTHAU. AUDREY HEPBURN. RICHARD BURTON. GALE STORM. BILL HEATON. INEZ ROBBINS. MAUREEN STAPLETON. GRACE JOHANSEN. HARRY COHEN. JANET FRANK. JILL CLAYBURGH. FREDDIE FIELDS. MARLON BRANDO. VINCENT CANBY. ROSE COHEN. GEORGE BARBER. GREGORY PECK. ORPHA AND WESLEY THEISEN. JACK SHAWN. GERALDINE PAGE. CHESTER HALL. WILLIAM EVERSON. MRS. CLARK. KERRY BASTENDORF. BILL BASTENDORF. RICHARD BROOKS. MARY ALICE HALL. TOM O'HORGAN. BEULAH KEATON. LEMUEL W. KEATON JR. ANNA KEATON. JACK N. HALL. DOROTHY DEANNE KEATON HALL.

ACKNOWLEDGMENTS

For Randy, Robin, and Dorrie, who shared the same mother but different experiences, and loved her their way. For my dear friends who read my words, and Mother's too: Carol Kane, Kathryn Grody Patinkin, and Stephen Shadley. For the valiant transcribers who saw scribble and made sentences: Jean Heaton, Arlene Smukler, and Saundra Schaffer. For Jean Stein, who gave me Bill Clegg . . . who in turn gave me David Ebershoff. For Joe Kelly, Bill Robinson, and Carolyn Barber, who supported me in my varied interests throughout the years. For Dr. Leo Rangell, who stuck with me in spite of my endless repetitions. For Susie Becker, Daniel Wolf, Larry McMurtry, Ann Carlson, Marvin Heiferman, Richard Pinter, Jonathan Gale, Sarah Paulsen, Nancy Meyers, Mary Sue and Josh Schweitzer, Alice Ann Wilson, Dr. Keith Agre, Debbie Durand, and Ronen Stromberg. For my darling companions, Josie, Red, Sweetie, and, last but not least, Emmie, and Dixie, our pet rat. For Woody Allen, Warren Beatty, Al Pacino, and Bill Bastendorf, who wrote so well. For Michael Gendler and Brian Fortman for getting the deal done. For Emily Blass and her designing eye. For Nick Reid's beautiful photographs of Mother's journals. For Eric Azra, who saved the documents I erased by mistake. To the team at Random House for actually publishing *Then Again,* including Gina Centrello, Susan Kamil, Sally Marvin, and David's assistant, Clare Swanson. For Anne Mayer, Susana Dionicio, and Irma Flores, who dearly cared for Mom. For Dorothy's doctors: Dr. Jeffrey Cummings and Dr. Claudia Kawas. If you'd like to make a donation to the Mary S. Easton Center for Alzheimer's Disease Research at UCLA, please visit www.eastonad.ucla.edu.

PHOTOGRAPHY and ARTWORK CAPTIONS and CREDITS

Opening photo spread © Annie Leibovitz,
courtesy of the artist

First Color Insert

Dorothy Hall's journals. PHOTO: NICK REID
Scrapbook of Diane Keaton, by Dorothy Hall. PHOTO:
   NICK REID
Page from Diane Keaton's scrapbook, by Dorothy Hall.
   PHOTO: NICK REID
Interiors of Dorothy's journals. PHOTO: NICK REID
Father and Daughters, collage by Dorothy Hall. PHOTO:
   NICK REID
Spines of Dorothy's journals. PHOTO: NICK REID

Black-and-White Insert

Diane as a child. PHOTO: DOROTHY HALL

Jack Hall.

Dorothy Hall and Diane as a baby.

Randy Hall. PHOTO: DOROTHY HALL

Robin (standing) and Dorrie Hall. PHOTO: DOROTHY HALL

Diane and Woody Allen. PHOTO: DOROTHY HALL

Diane as a young adult. PHOTO: FREDERIC OHRINGER

Diane close-up. PHOTO: SMP/GLOBE PHOTOS, INC.

Diane in a suit. PHOTO: © GARY LEWIS/CAMERAPRESS/
  RETNA LTD, USA

Diane and Dorothy Hall. PHOTO: JACK HALL

Diane with hands by head. PHOTO: DOROTHY HALL

Warren Beatty. PHOTO: COURTESY OF PARAMOUNT PICTURES.
  Heaven Can Wait copyright 1979 by Paramount Pictures
  Corporation. All rights reserved.

Al Pacino on the set. PHOTO: COURTESY OF PARAMOUNT
  PICTURES. *The Godfather: Part III* copyright 1990 by
  Paramount Pictures Corporation. All rights reserved.

Duke and Dexter Keaton. PHOTO: JULIA DEAN

Diane with Duke and Dexter. PHOTO: RUVEN AFANADOR

Diane with pearls. PHOTO: MICHEL COMTE

Second Color Insert

Ear, collage by Dorothy Hall. PHOTO: NICK REID

Honor Thy Self, collage by Dorothy Hall. PHOTO: NICK
  REID

Woman with Hand on Breast, collage by Dorothy Hall.
  PHOTO: NICK REID

THINK, found pinned up on Dorothy Hall's bulletin
board. PHOTO: NICK REID

"Who Says You Haven't Got a Chance?" collage by
Dorothy Hall. PHOTO: NICK REID

Legs, collage by Dorothy Hall. PHOTO: NICK REID

Or Not to Be, collage by Dorothy Hall. PHOTO: NICK REID

ABOUT THE AUTHOR

DIANE KEATON has starred in some of the most memorable movies of the past forty years, including the *Godfather* trilogy, *Annie Hall, Manhattan, Reds, Baby Boom, The First Wives Club,* and *Something's Gotta Give.* Her many awards include the Golden Globe and the Academy Award. Keaton lives with her daughter and son in Los Angeles.

ABOUT THE TYPE

This book was set in Sabon, a typeface designed by the well-known German typographer Jan Tschichold (1902–74). Sabon's design is based on the original letterforms of Claude Garamond and was created specifically to be used for three sources: foundry type for hand composition, Linotype, and Monotype. Tschichold named his typeface for the famous Frankfurt typefounder Jacques Sabon, who died in 1580.